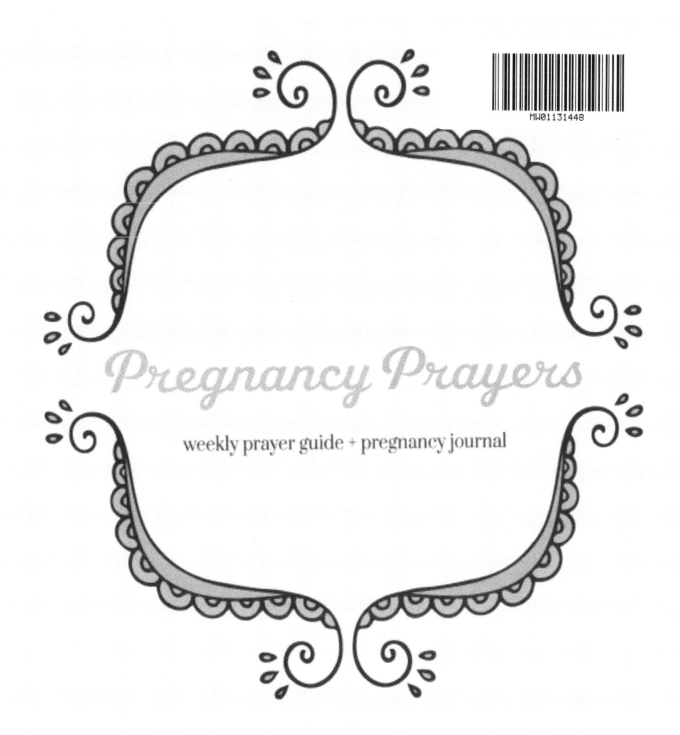

Pregnancy Prayers

weekly prayer guide + pregnancy journal

by ASHLEY SIMS

It is critical that we speak words of life and pray over our unborn babies. The world tells us they are not valuable but the word of God says differently.

Psalm 139:13-15 NLT

13 You made all the delicate, inner parts of my body
and knit me together in my mother's womb.
14 Thank you for making me so wonderfully complex!
Your workmanship is marvelous—how well I know it.
15 You watched me as I was being formed in utter seclusion,
as I was woven together in the dark of the womb.

I encourage all expectant mothers to read and enjoy *Pregnancy Prayers.*

Gloria Copeland

Gloria Copeland

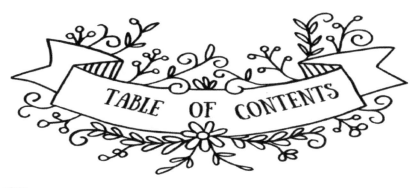

TABLE OF CONTENTS

MY PERSONAL
TESTIMONY

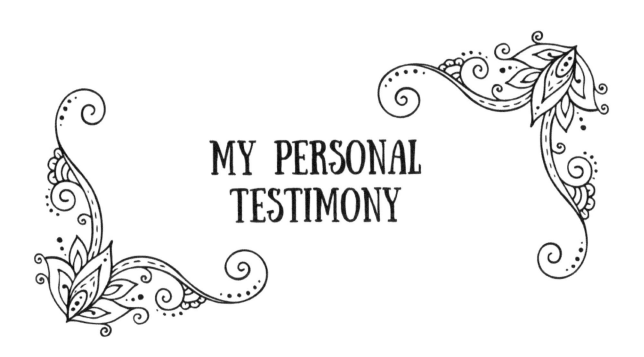

It was during my pregnancy with our second baby that I began writing the Pregnancy Prayers app. I kept searching for the "right" words to pray over our sweet baby. I never felt any fear or anxiety about our first pregnancy, but something was different this time. Maybe it was that I knew too much of what could go wrong. Several of my friends had just had miscarriages and one of our close friends had just received the news that their baby had no chance of survival out of the womb. With all the "what ifs" rolling around in my brain, I needed to know what to pray to help bring me peace. I desperately wanted to find an app that could send me a daily reminder to pray for my baby and, better yet, tell me what to pray too. When I couldn't find one, I decided to write an app based on the baby's weekly development, and most importantly, the Word of God.

A couple of months into my pregnancy things were going well until I had a major bleed, and due to my friends' experiences of miscarriages, I assumed I was having one too. I tried not to panic, I really did, but let's be honest; I was completely terrified I would lose my baby too. After a quick trip to the doctor, I discovered that I had only ruptured a vessel in my uterus due to too much exercise. Baby Sims was healthy and growing just as she should. I was no longer allowed to exercise, which just gave me more time to write my app. The next several weeks were nothing but smooth sailing in my pregnancy. We were eagerly counting down the time until we could find out the gender of our baby. I had set a goal to finish writing the app before I delivered, and I was writing every chance I could get. On the day of my 29th birthday my husband, Paul, and I went to find out our sweet baby's gender. We both were hoping for a girl and our son, Cooper, had been telling everyone he was having a sister from the moment he found out I was pregnant. True to form, Cooper was right! We were having a little girl, Scarlett Elizabeth! We left the ultrasound ready to surprise our families with the wonderful news.

Just a few short days later, we packed up and headed to the middle of nowhere in Colorado with my husband's family for a week. This meant no cellphone reception, lots of fishing for the boys, and lots of time to write for this momma! Halfway through our trip, we headed into town to explore. This was our first time in several days to have cellphone reception. It was in Pagosa Springs, Colorado, that we heard from the doctor that they found more than just our baby's gender at our last ultrasound. The nurse at our doctor's office informed me that Scarlett had two choroid plexus cysts on her brain and we needed to get back to see a specialist for specialized scans immediately.

Let me tell you, don't google choroid plexus cysts. There are two options: 1. These cysts are a sign that your baby has trisomy 18 and will most likely be born as a stillborn if they make it to birth. 2. The cysts mean nothing and dissolve off the baby's brain before they are born and you never knew they were there. One word... sobbing. In the middle of a Mexican food restaurant, with all my husband's family, I sobbed the tears of a mother who was afraid she would lose her baby. I've seen my extremely macho husband shed one tear since I have known him and it was when he thought he might lose his little princess. I had time to call my mom and tell her the news, and thankfully my Mother is a woman of prayer. She prayed with me over Scarlett and we began to thank God, in faith, for our healthy baby girl. After that, we headed back to the electronics' free silence of mother nature. Nobody knew what to say, so Paul and I decided we just wouldn't talk about it until we got back to Fort Worth to find out what the specialist saw in our next ultrasound. Looking back now, I can see that this was one of the best decisions we made. Neither one of us wanted to speak negatively about what could go wrong with Scarlett, so we just prayed for the best results to show up on the scans. We packed up the next morning and headed back home. At our sonogram with the specialist, she did not see any other markers for trisomy 18. This meant that Scarlett just had cysts on her brain that would dissolve on their own before she was born.

Now, I can see God knew Scarlett would need me to be praying for her. He knew Scarlett needed me to stand in the gap for her and be in continuous prayer for her health and development. This is why I am so passionate about the Pregnancy Prayers app and now the Pregnancy Prayers book. I will forever be grateful that the Holy Spirit kept bringing up the importance of praying for Scarlett to my heart. I am thankful that I wrote all the prayers while I was pregnant with her, and it is my hope that now these prayers will bring peace and guidance to other expectant parents.

I pray that the content in this book guides your prayer life for your baby and encourages you in your walk with the Lord.

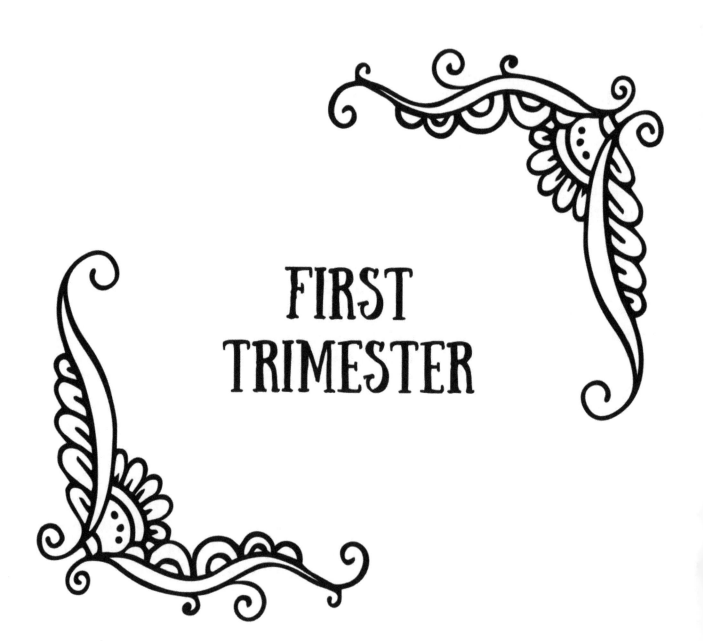

FIRST
TRIMESTER

The joy
of the LORD
is my
STRENGTH.
Nehemiah 8:10

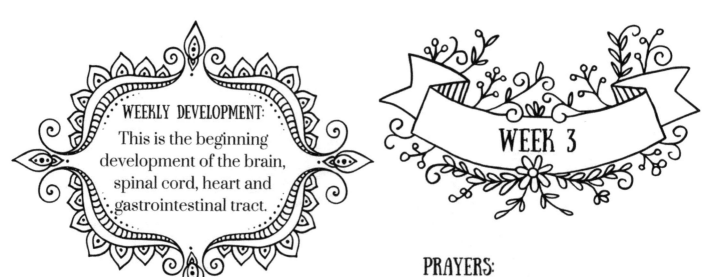

WEEKLY DEVELOPMENT: This is the beginning development of the brain, spinal cord, heart and gastrointestinal tract.

WEEK 3

PRAYERS:
DEAR LORD, I THANK YOU FOR THE OPPORTUNITY TO BE FRUITFUL AND MULTIPLY. I ASK FOR AN EASY PREGNANCY RIGHT FROM THE START.

FATHER GOD, I PRAY OVER THE MIRACLE OCCURRING IN MY BODY RIGHT NOW. I KNOW THIS BABY IS JUST A TINY SPECK, BUT I THANK YOU FOR HIM.

LORD, I PRAY OVER THE DEVELOPMENT OF THE BABY'S BRAIN AND SPINAL CORD. I ASK YOU TO WATCH OVER THE DEVELOPMENT AND KEEP MY BABY SAFE.

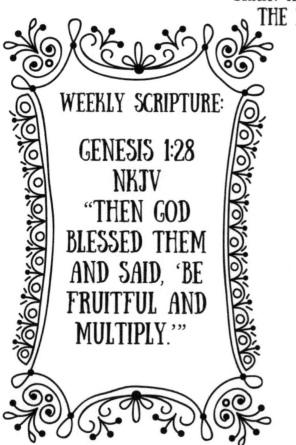

WEEKLY SCRIPTURE:

GENESIS 1:28 NKJV "THEN GOD BLESSED THEM AND SAID, 'BE FRUITFUL AND MULTIPLY.'"

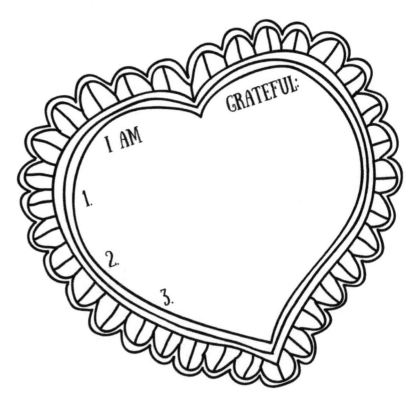

I AM GRATEFUL:

1.

2.

3.

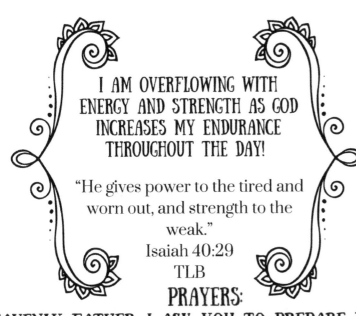

I AM OVERFLOWING WITH ENERGY AND STRENGTH AS GOD INCREASES MY ENDURANCE THROUGHOUT THE DAY!

"He gives power to the tired and worn out, and strength to the weak."
Isaiah 40:29
TLB

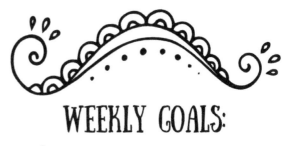

WEEKLY GOALS:

1.

2.

3.

PRAYERS:

HEAVENLY FATHER, I ASK YOU TO PREPARE MY BODY FOR PREGNANCY, AND I ASK THAT ALL OF MY HORMONE LEVELS WILL BE AT EXACTLY THE RIGHT PLACES TO CARRY THIS MIRACLE.

LORD GOD, I PRAY OVER THE GASTROINTESTINAL TRACT IN THIS BABY, AND I ASK THAT IT NEVER HAVE PROBLEMS IN THE WOMB OR AFTER DELIVERY.

DEAR GOD, I PRAY OVER THE MIRACLE THAT IS MY BABY'S HEART. IT IS ABSOLUTELY AMAZING THAT SOMETHING SO TINY CAN HAVE BODY PARTS THAT ARE SO INTRICATE. I PRAY THAT THIS HEART WILL GROW STRONG AND MIGHTY.

MY PRAYERS:

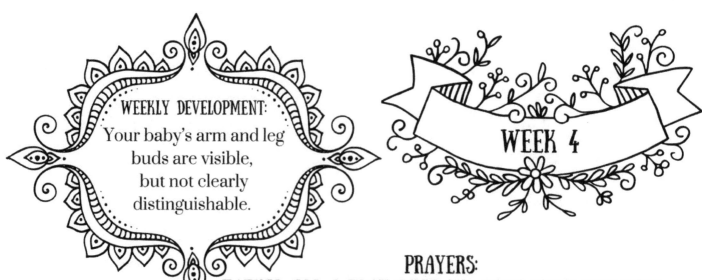

WEEKLY DEVELOPMENT:
Your baby's arm and leg buds are visible, but not clearly distinguishable.

WEEK 4

PRAYERS:
FATHER GOD, I PRAY OVER MY BODY THAT YOU WILL PREPARE IT TO CARRY THIS BABY TO FULL TERM.

LORD, I THANK YOU FOR THIS GROWING BABY. I PRAY OVER THE GROWING LEG BUDS, THAT THEY WILL GROW STRAIGHT AND STRONG.

GOD, IN THIS BEGINNING STAGE OF PREGNANCY, I THANK YOU FOR YOUR JOY AND THAT I WILL ENJOY THIS PREGNANCY.

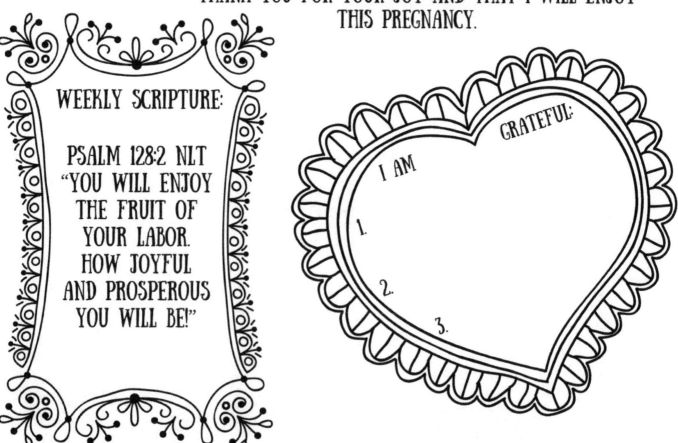

WEEKLY SCRIPTURE:

PSALM 128:2 NLT
"YOU WILL ENJOY THE FRUIT OF YOUR LABOR. HOW JOYFUL AND PROSPEROUS YOU WILL BE!"

I AM GRATEFUL:
1.
2.
3.

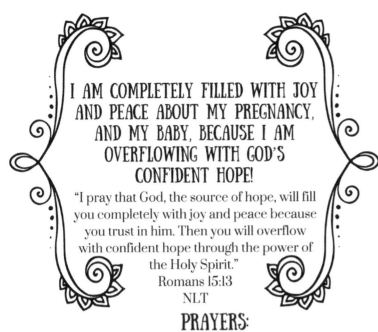

I AM COMPLETELY FILLED WITH JOY AND PEACE ABOUT MY PREGNANCY, AND MY BABY, BECAUSE I AM OVERFLOWING WITH GOD'S CONFIDENT HOPE!

"I pray that God, the source of hope, will fill you completely with joy and peace because you trust in him. Then you will overflow with confident hope through the power of the Holy Spirit."
Romans 15:13
NLT

WEEKLY GOALS:

1.

2.

3.

PRAYERS:

DEAR LORD, I PRAY OVER THE ARM BUDS THAT ARE FORMING ON MY BABY. I PRAY THEY WILL GROW, AND THAT EVERY MUSCLE, JOINT AND BONE WILL COME TOGETHER PERFECTLY.

DEAR GOD, BLESS THIS TINY BABY TODAY. I PRAY OVER THE HEALTHY ORGANS THAT ARE CONTINUING TO DEVELOP, AND I ASK YOU TO KEEP WATCH OVER MY BABY EVERY DAY.

HEAVENLY FATHER, I CONTINUE TO PRAY OVER MY BODY AND MY HORMONE LEVELS. I PRAY THEY WILL CONTINUE TO STAY AT THE LEVELS NEEDED TO KEEP MY BODY AS A PERFECT HOME FOR THIS GROWING BABY.

MY PRAYERS:

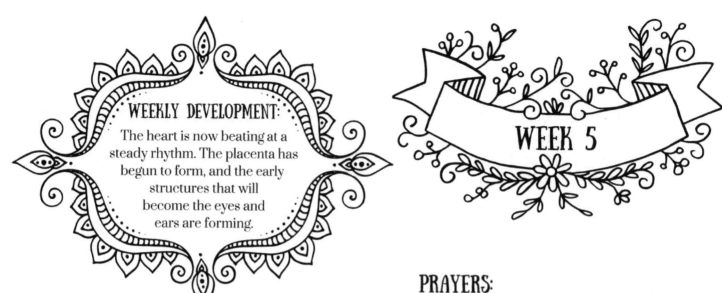

WEEKLY DEVELOPMENT:
The heart is now beating at a steady rhythm. The placenta has begun to form, and the early structures that will become the eyes and ears are forming.

WEEK 5

PRAYERS:
LORD GOD, I PRAY OVER THE FORMING PLACENTA. I THANK YOU THAT IT WILL HAVE THE ABILITY TO FULLY NOURISH MY BABY UNTIL HE IS DEVELOPED TO FULL TERM.

TODAY I AM SO THANKFUL THAT MY BABY HAS A STEADY HEARTBEAT. I PRAY THIS PREGNANCY WILL BE BLESSED AND WILL NOT RESULT IN A MISCARRIAGE.

LORD, I ASK YOU FOR WISDOM TODAY. GIVE ME THE WISDOM TO KNOW HOW TO MAKE MY BODY A PERFECT PLACE TO GROW THIS CHILD.

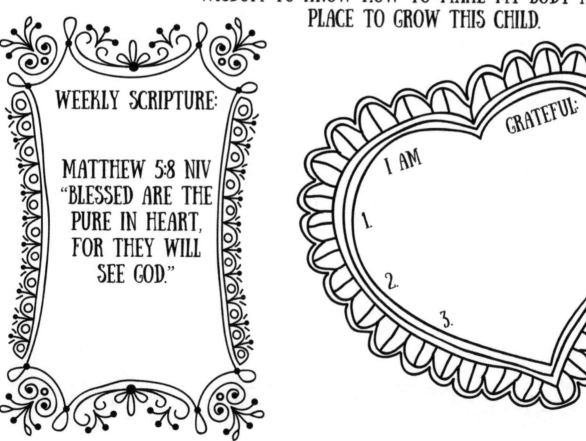

WEEKLY SCRIPTURE:

MATTHEW 5:8 NIV
"BLESSED ARE THE PURE IN HEART, FOR THEY WILL SEE GOD."

I AM GRATEFUL:
1.
2.
3.

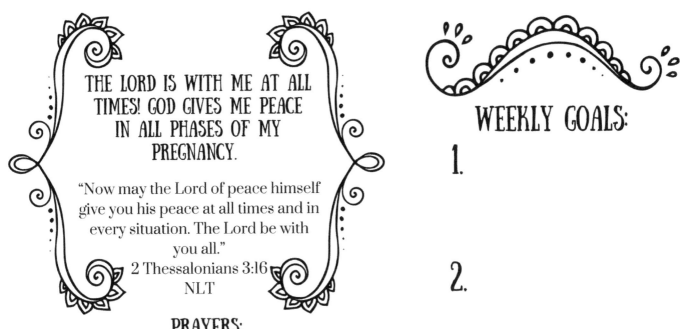

THE LORD IS WITH ME AT ALL TIMES! GOD GIVES ME PEACE IN ALL PHASES OF MY PREGNANCY.

"Now may the Lord of peace himself give you his peace at all times and in every situation. The Lord be with you all."
2 Thessalonians 3:16
NLT

WEEKLY GOALS:

1.

2.

3.

PRAYERS:
HEAVENLY FATHER, I ASK YOU TO BLESS THE LITTLE EARS THAT ARE FORMING ON MY BABY. I PRAY THEY WILL FUNCTION FULLY FROM THE MOMENT MY BABY IS BORN.

FATHER GOD, I THANK YOU FOR A BABY WHO IS PURE IN HEART. I PRAY MY CHILD WILL ALWAYS HAVE A PURE HEART, AND THAT HE WILL KNOW YOU.

LORD, I THANK YOU FOR GIVING ME THE STRENGTH AND ENERGY TO CARRY THIS BABY. I ASK YOU TO BLESS MY BODY AS IT BEGINS TO CARRY AND PRODUCE THIS MIRACLE.

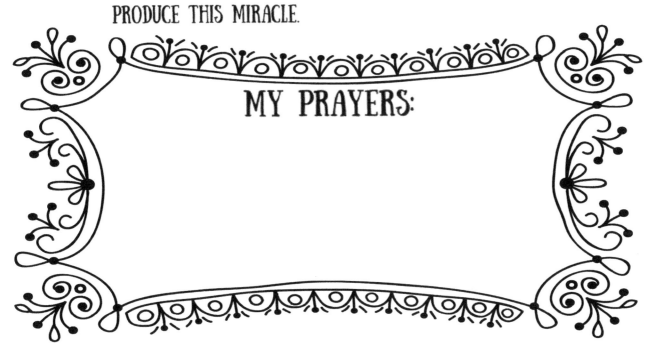

MY PRAYERS:

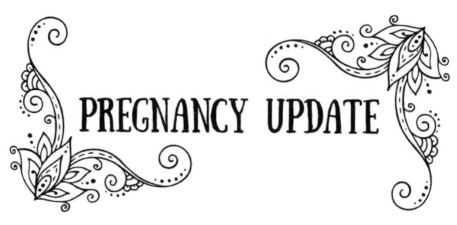

PREGNANCY UPDATE

EMOTIONS I'M FEELING:

_____
_____
_____
_____

PREGNANCY SYMPTOMS:

_____
_____
_____
_____

FOODS:

CAN'T GET ENOUGH:

_____
_____
_____

CAN'T STAND:

_____
_____
_____

FAVORITE PREGNANCY OUTFIT:

_____
_____
_____
_____

NOTES TO MY BABY:

_____
_____
_____
_____

BABY OR BUMP PICTURE

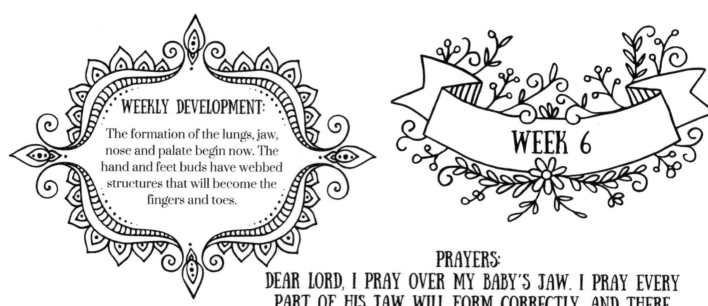

WEEKLY DEVELOPMENT:

The formation of the lungs, jaw, nose and palate begin now. The hand and feet buds have webbed structures that will become the fingers and toes.

WEEK 6

PRAYERS:

DEAR LORD, I PRAY OVER MY BABY'S JAW. I PRAY EVERY PART OF HIS JAW WILL FORM CORRECTLY, AND THERE WILL BE NO PROBLEMS AT ANY POINT WITH MY BABY'S SWEET FACE.

FATHER GOD, I THANK YOU FOR GIVING MY CHILD THE BREATH OF LIFE AND FILLING HIS LUNGS WITH YOU. I ASK THAT YOUR PRESENCE BE WITH THIS CHILD ALL THE DAYS OF HIS LIFE.

DEAR GOD, TODAY I PRAY OVER THE FORMATION OF MY CHILD'S PALATE. I SPEAK AGAINST ANY IRREGULARITIES IN HIS PALATE. I BELIEVE IT WILL FORM PERFECTLY AND WHOLE IN JESUS' NAME.

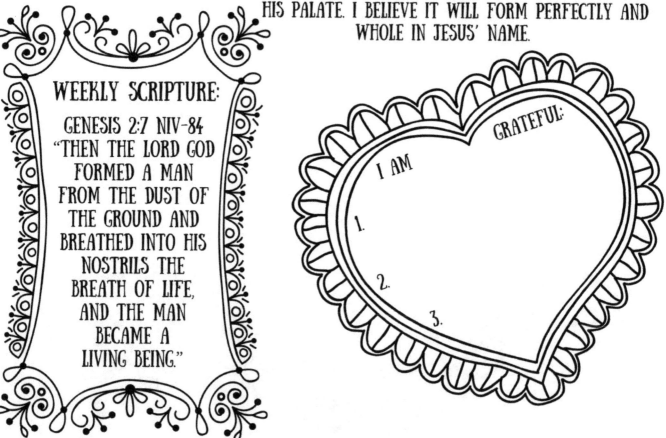

WEEKLY SCRIPTURE:

GENESIS 2:7 NIV-84
"THEN THE LORD GOD FORMED A MAN FROM THE DUST OF THE GROUND AND BREATHED INTO HIS NOSTRILS THE BREATH OF LIFE, AND THE MAN BECAME A LIVING BEING."

I AM GRATEFUL:

1.

2.

3.

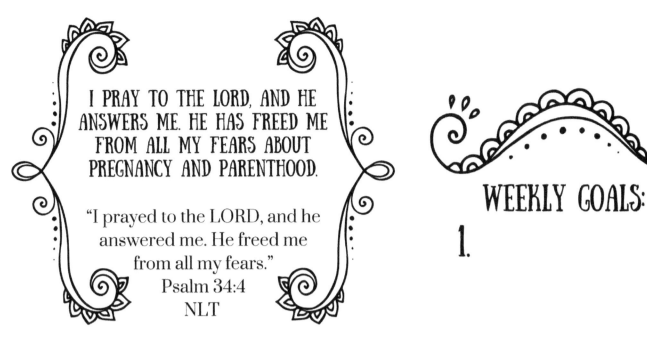

I PRAY TO THE LORD, AND HE ANSWERS ME. HE HAS FREED ME FROM ALL MY FEARS ABOUT PREGNANCY AND PARENTHOOD.

"I prayed to the LORD, and he answered me. He freed me from all my fears."
Psalm 34:4
NLT

WEEKLY GOALS:

1.

2.

3.

PRAYERS:
THANK YOU, LORD, FOR MY BABY'S PRECIOUS FEET! I SPEAK OVER HIS FEET, THAT THEY WILL ALWAYS WALK DOWN THE CORRECT PATH, AND THAT THIS BABY'S STEPS ARE ORDERED BY YOU.

DEAR HEAVENLY FATHER, I THANK YOU FOR THE LITTLE HANDS THAT ARE BEGINNING TO FORM. I PRAY EVERY BONE AND EVERY LIGAMENT WILL FORM PROPERLY, AND WHATEVER THIS CHILD SETS HIS HAND TO DO WILL PROSPER.

TODAY I ASK FOR THE ENERGY AND ABILITY TO CONTINUE TO CARRY THIS CHILD. I PRAY YOU WILL HELP MY BODY TO BRING THIS BABY TO FULL TERM SUCCESSFULLY.

MY PRAYERS:

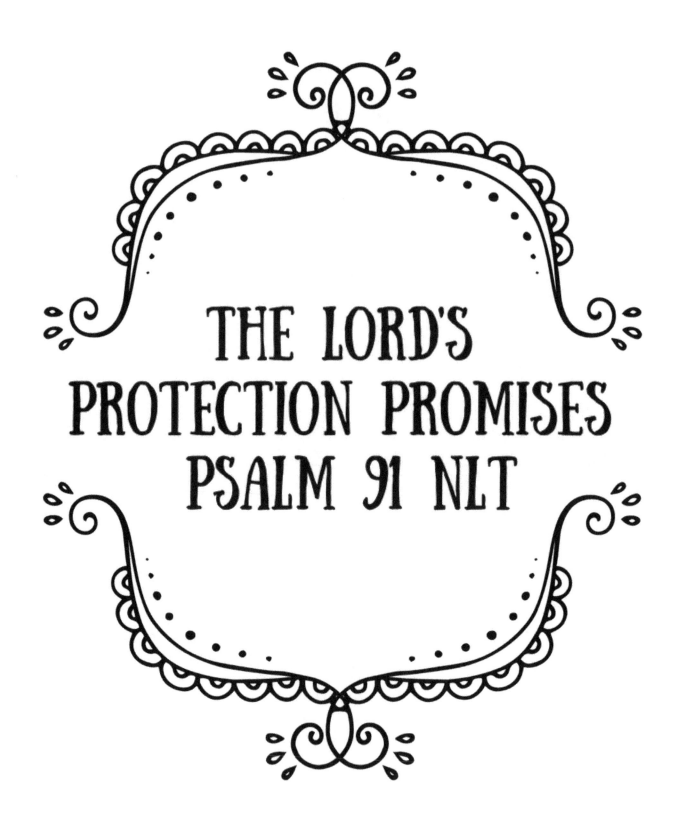

THE LORD'S
PROTECTION PROMISES
PSALM 91 NLT

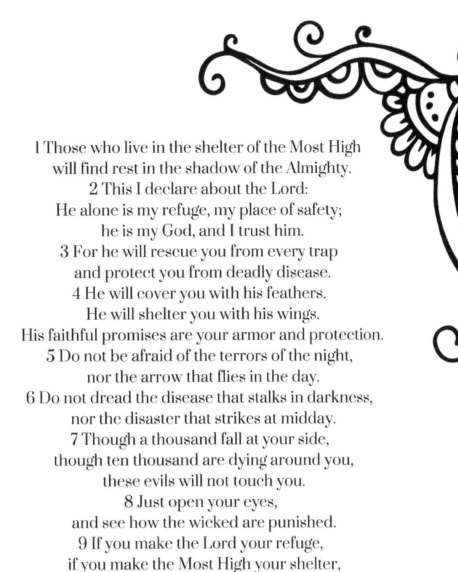

1 Those who live in the shelter of the Most High
will find rest in the shadow of the Almighty.
2 This I declare about the Lord:
He alone is my refuge, my place of safety;
he is my God, and I trust him.
3 For he will rescue you from every trap
and protect you from deadly disease.
4 He will cover you with his feathers.
He will shelter you with his wings.
His faithful promises are your armor and protection.
5 Do not be afraid of the terrors of the night,
nor the arrow that flies in the day.
6 Do not dread the disease that stalks in darkness,
nor the disaster that strikes at midday.
7 Though a thousand fall at your side,
though ten thousand are dying around you,
these evils will not touch you.
8 Just open your eyes,
and see how the wicked are punished.
9 If you make the Lord your refuge,
if you make the Most High your shelter,
10 no evil will conquer you;
no plague will come near your home.
11 For he will order his angels
to protect you wherever you go.
12 They will hold you up with their hands
so you won't even hurt your foot on a stone.
13 You will trample upon lions and cobras;
you will crush fierce lions and serpents under your feet!
14 The Lord says, "I will rescue those who love me.
I will protect those who trust in my name.
15 When they call on me, I will answer;
I will be with them in trouble.
I will rescue and honor them.
16 I will reward them with a long life
and give them my salvation."

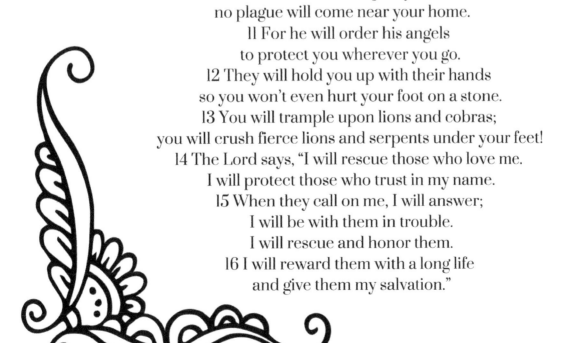

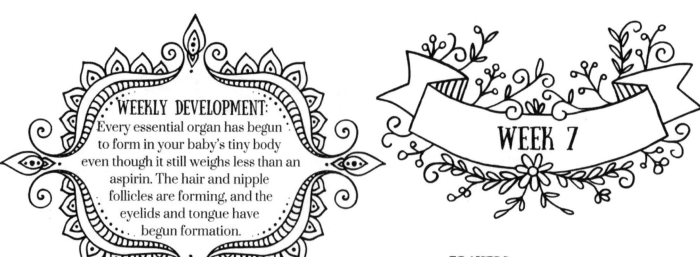

WEEKLY DEVELOPMENT:
Every essential organ has begun to form in your baby's tiny body even though it still weighs less than an aspirin. The hair and nipple follicles are forming, and the eyelids and tongue have begun formation.

WEEK 7

PRAYERS:

DEAR GOD, I THANK YOU FOR EVERY WONDROUS WORK YOU ARE DOING IN MY BABY THIS WEEK. I PRAY OVER THE TINY ORGANS THAT ARE BEGINNING TO DEVELOP AND THAT EACH AND EVERY ONE WILL FULFILL ITS ROLE WITHIN THIS BODY FLAWLESSLY.

DEAR HEAVENLY FATHER, I THANK YOU THAT EVEN THOUGH MY CHILD IS STILL SO TINY AND NEW, HE IS STILL IMPORTANT ENOUGH TO YOU THAT YOU KNOW THE NUMBER OF HAIRS ON HIS HEAD, AND HE WILL ALWAYS BE IMPORTANT TO YOU.

DEAR LORD, I PRAY OVER MY BABY'S FORMING TONGUE. THIS TONGUE WILL FORM PERFECTLY AND WILL FOREVER SPEAK OF LOVE FOR YOU.

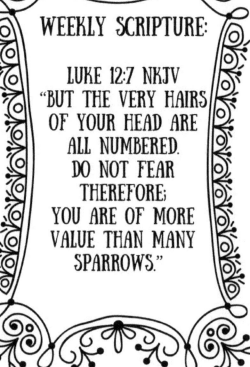

WEEKLY SCRIPTURE:

LUKE 12:7 NKJV
"BUT THE VERY HAIRS OF YOUR HEAD ARE ALL NUMBERED. DO NOT FEAR THEREFORE; YOU ARE OF MORE VALUE THAN MANY SPARROWS."

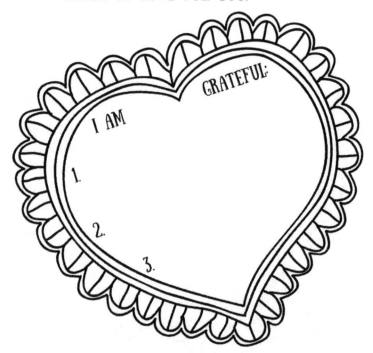

I AM GRATEFUL:

1.

2.

3.

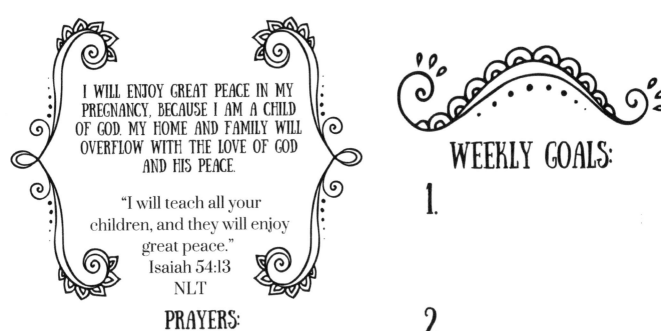

I WILL ENJOY GREAT PEACE IN MY PREGNANCY, BECAUSE I AM A CHILD OF GOD. MY HOME AND FAMILY WILL OVERFLOW WITH THE LOVE OF GOD AND HIS PEACE.

"I will teach all your children, and they will enjoy great peace."
Isaiah 54:13
NLT

WEEKLY GOALS:

1.

2.

3.

PRAYERS:

LORD, TODAY I THANK YOU THAT I HAVE THE STRENGTH TO CARRY THIS BABY! I BELIEVE I HAVE THE ENERGY AND ABILITY TO HAVE A GREAT PREGNANCY!

FATHER GOD, I PRAY OVER THIS TINY BABY AND THAT EVEN THOUGH HE IS TINY, HE IS MIGHTY AND STRONG.

LORD, I ASK YOU TO HELP ME NOT TO BE FEARFUL IN THIS CRUCIAL PART OF PREGNANCY. I TRUST THAT YOU HAVE A PERFECT PLAN FOR THIS PREGNANCY.

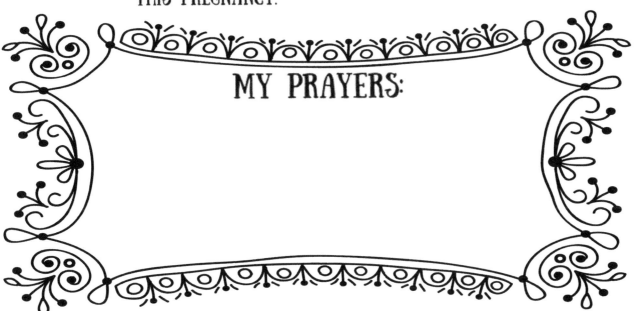

MY PRAYERS:

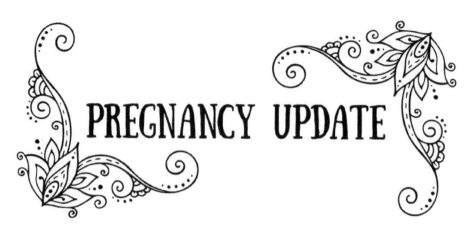

PREGNANCY UPDATE

EMOTIONS I'M FEELING:

_____
_____
_____
_____

PREGNANCY SYMPTOMS:

_____
_____
_____
_____

FOODS:

CAN'T GET ENOUGH:

_____
_____
_____

CAN'T STAND:

_____
_____

FAVORITE PREGNANCY OUTFIT:

_____
_____
_____
_____

NOTES TO MY BABY:

_____
_____
_____
_____

BABY OR BUMP
PICTURE

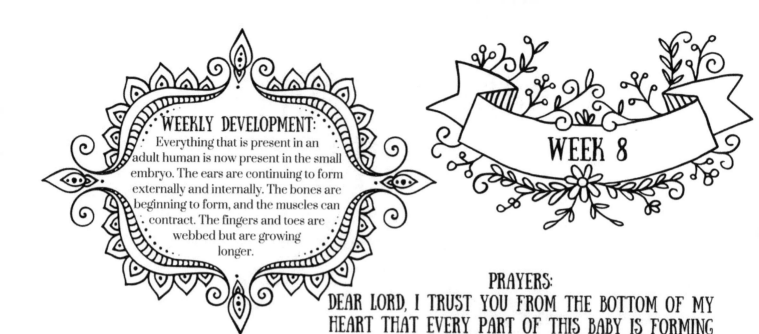

WEEKLY DEVELOPMENT:
Everything that is present in an adult human is now present in the small embryo. The ears are continuing to form externally and internally. The bones are beginning to form, and the muscles can contract. The fingers and toes are webbed but are growing longer.

WEEK 8

PRAYERS:
DEAR LORD, I TRUST YOU FROM THE BOTTOM OF MY HEART THAT EVERY PART OF THIS BABY IS FORMING CORRECTLY. I THANK YOU FOR THE PLAN YOU HAVE ESTABLISHED FOR THIS CHILD.

FATHER GOD, I PRAY OVER THIS BABY'S FORMING EARS, THAT THEY WILL HEAR PERFECTLY, AND THEY WILL FORM CORRECTLY INTERNALLY AND EXTERNALLY.

HEAVENLY FATHER, I ASK THAT NOT ONLY DOES MY CHILD HAVE EARS TO HEAR, BUT ALSO EARS TO HEAR YOUR VOICE, SO THAT YOU CAN LEAD HIM ON THE PATH YOU HAVE PLANNED FOR HIM.

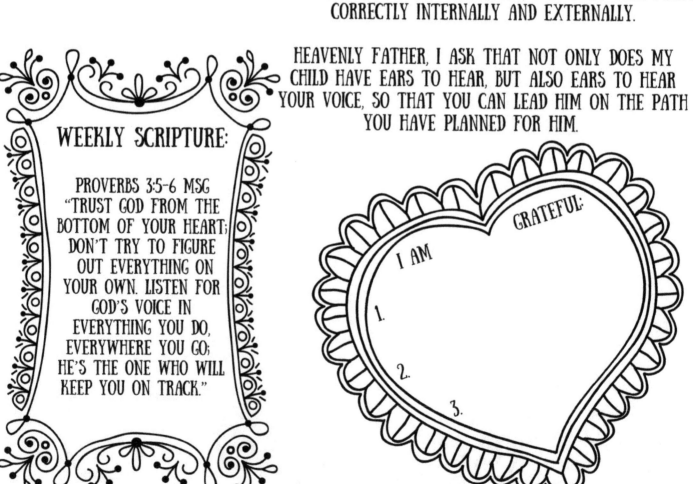

WEEKLY SCRIPTURE:

PROVERBS 3:5-6 MSG
"TRUST GOD FROM THE BOTTOM OF YOUR HEART; DON'T TRY TO FIGURE OUT EVERYTHING ON YOUR OWN. LISTEN FOR GOD'S VOICE IN EVERYTHING YOU DO, EVERYWHERE YOU GO; HE'S THE ONE WHO WILL KEEP YOU ON TRACK."

I AM   GRATEFUL:
1.
2.
3.

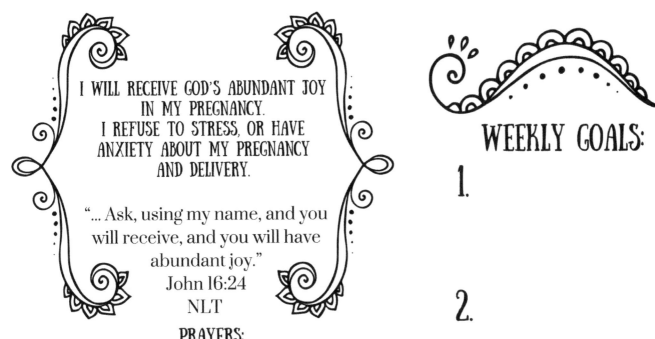

I WILL RECEIVE GOD'S ABUNDANT JOY
IN MY PREGNANCY.
I REFUSE TO STRESS, OR HAVE
ANXIETY ABOUT MY PREGNANCY
AND DELIVERY.

"... Ask, using my name, and you
will receive, and you will have
abundant joy."
John 16:24
NLT

PRAYERS:

TODAY, I THANK YOU FOR MY BABY'S PRECIOUS WEBBED FINGERS AND TOES. I ASK YOU TO BLESS EACH FINGER AND EACH TOE AND ALLOW THEM TO GROW AS THEY SHOULD.

DEAR GOD, I THANK YOU FOR THE MIRACLE THAT IS GROWING INSIDE ME. IT IS AN ABSOLUTE WONDER THAT THIS TINY BEING HAS EVERY ORGAN AND BODY PART THAT A GROWN HUMAN HAS.

LORD, I ASK YOU TO WATCH OVER THE GROWTH OF THIS BABY'S BONES AND THAT FROM THE TOP OF HIS TINY HEAD TO THE BOTTOM OF HIS FEET, EVERY BONE WILL FORM CORRECTLY AND BE STRONG AND NEVER BRITTLE.

WEEKLY GOALS:

1.

2.

3.

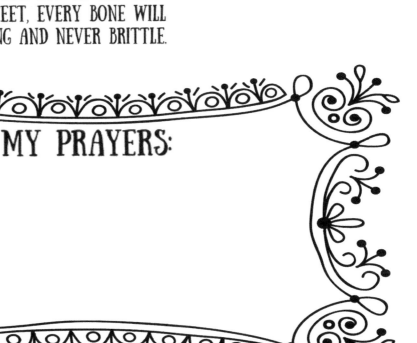

MY PRAYERS:

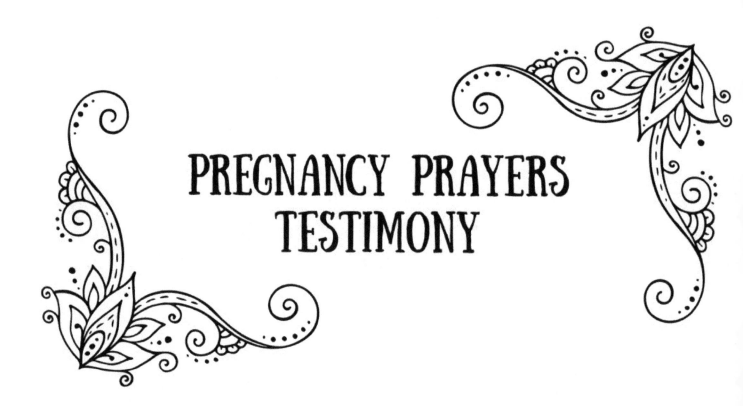

PREGNANCY PRAYERS
TESTIMONY

The Pregnancy Prayers app has been a true blessing to have through my pregnancy! A tricky talented woman of God put together just the prayers a mother needs to read during each point in pregnancy!

Thank you, Ashley Sims, for doing such a great job on Pregnancy Prayers!
— Courtney

Download the Pregnancy Prayers app in iTunes and the Google Play stores.

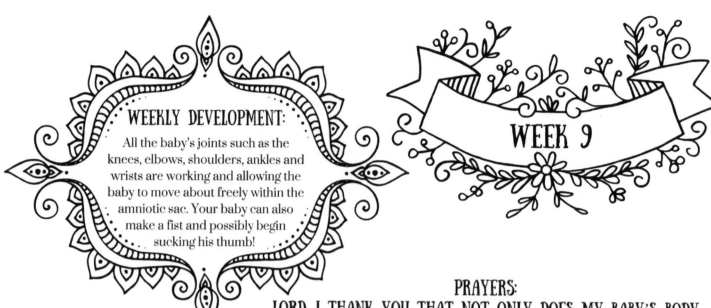

WEEKLY DEVELOPMENT:

All the baby's joints such as the knees, elbows, shoulders, ankles and wrists are working and allowing the baby to move about freely within the amniotic sac. Your baby can also make a fist and possibly begin sucking his thumb!

WEEK 9

PRAYERS:

LORD, I THANK YOU THAT NOT ONLY DOES MY BABY'S BODY GLOW WITH HEALTH, BUT MY BODY DOES TOO. I BELIEVE I AM THE PERFECT VESSEL TO CARRY THIS BABY, AND I WILL GLOW WITH HEALTH THROUGH THIS WHOLE PREGNANCY.

DEAR GOD, I BELIEVE MY SWEET BABY'S BONES VIBRATE WITH LIFE! I SPEAK OVER EVERY BONE AND JOINT IN HIS BODY AND BELIEVE EACH ONE WILL FUNCTION CORRECTLY AND WITHOUT PAIN ALL THE DAYS OF THIS BABY'S LIFE.

DEAR HEAVENLY FATHER, I PRAY FOR MY BABY'S MOVEMENTS IN MY WOMB AND THAT STARTING NOW, AND EVERY DAY THAT FOLLOWS, EVERY MOVE HE MAKES IS ORDERED OF YOU.

WEEKLY SCRIPTURE:

PROVERBS 3:8-9 MSG "YOUR BODY WILL GLOW WITH HEALTH, YOUR VERY BONES WILL VIBRATE WITH LIFE! HONOR GOD WITH EVERYTHING YOU OWN; GIVE HIM THE FIRST AND THE BEST."

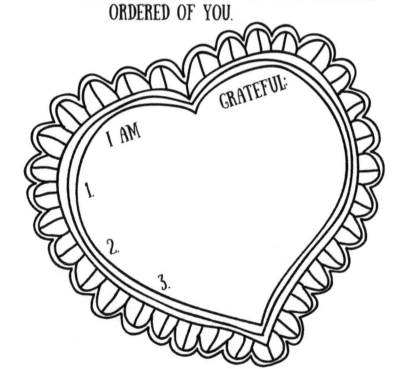

I AM GRATEFUL:

1.

2.

3.

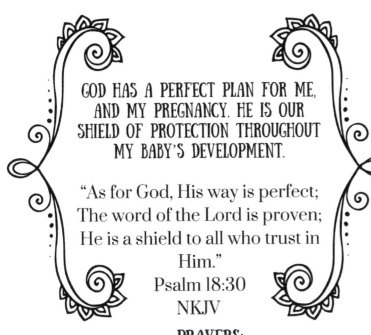

GOD HAS A PERFECT PLAN FOR ME, AND MY PREGNANCY. HE IS OUR SHIELD OF PROTECTION THROUGHOUT MY BABY'S DEVELOPMENT.

"As for God, His way is perfect; The word of the Lord is proven; He is a shield to all who trust in Him."
Psalm 18:30
NKJV

PRAYERS:

LORD, TODAY I GIVE YOU MY BEST. I SET OUT TO RAISE THIS BABY FOR YOU. I ASK YOU TO GIVE ME THE STRENGTH AND WISDOM TO BE AN INCREDIBLE PARENT TO THIS CHILD.

FATHER GOD, I PRAY OVER THE JOINTS THAT ARE FORMING IN MY BABY. I PRAY THEY WILL ALL DEVELOP AND GROW JUST AS THEY SHOULD TO ENSURE THAT MY CHILD DOES NOT HAVE JOINT ISSUES OUT OF THE WOMB.

DEAR LORD, I THANK YOU FOR THE MIRACLE THAT IS GROWING IN ME. IT IS AMAZING THAT MY BABY CAN ALREADY SUCK HIS THUMB! I PRAY THIS BABY WILL CONTINUE TO BE A SELF-SOOTHER AFTER DELIVERY.

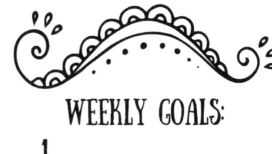

WEEKLY GOALS:

1.

2.

3.

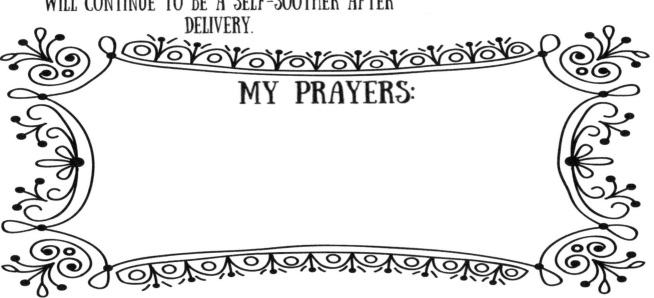

MY PRAYERS:

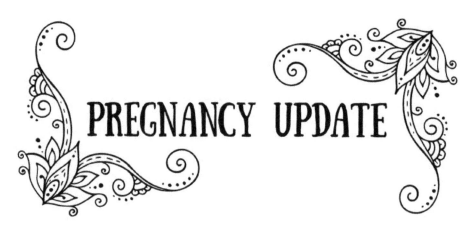

PREGNANCY UPDATE

EMOTIONS I'M FEELING:

_____
_____
_____
_____

PREGNANCY SYMPTOMS:

_____
_____
_____
_____

FOODS:

CAN'T GET ENOUGH:

_____
_____
_____

CAN'T STAND:

_____
_____
_____

FAVORITE PREGNANCY OUTFIT:

_____
_____
_____

NOTES TO MY BABY:

_____
_____
_____
_____

BABY OR BUMP
PICTURE

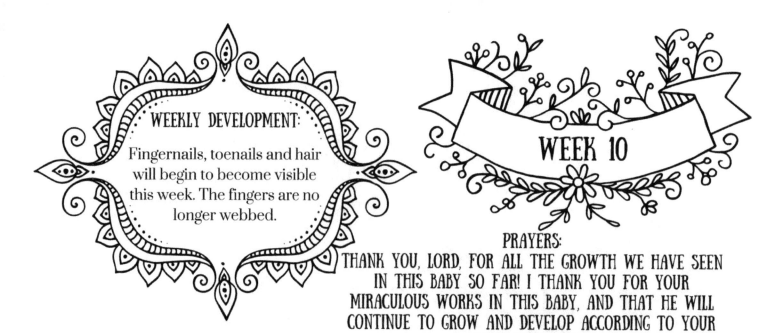

WEEKLY DEVELOPMENT:

Fingernails, toenails and hair will begin to become visible this week. The fingers are no longer webbed.

WEEK 10

PRAYERS:

THANK YOU, LORD, FOR ALL THE GROWTH WE HAVE SEEN IN THIS BABY SO FAR! I THANK YOU FOR YOUR MIRACULOUS WORKS IN THIS BABY, AND THAT HE WILL CONTINUE TO GROW AND DEVELOP ACCORDING TO YOUR PLAN EVERY DAY.

LORD GOD, TODAY I PRAY OVER THIS BABY'S NAILS AND HAIR. I KNOW THAT EVEN THOUGH THESE ARE MINOR THINGS TO SOME, THEY ARE JUST AS IMPORTANT TO YOU AS THEY ARE TO ME. I PRAY THEY GROW IN SEAMLESSLY AND WILL CONTINUE TO DEVELOP AS THIS CHILD GROWS AND MATURES THROUGHOUT HIS LIFE.

TODAY I PRAY OVER MY BABY'S FINGERS AND TOES THAT ARE BECOMING THEIR OWN EXTREMITIES AS THEY DETACH FROM THEIR WEBBED FORM. I SPEAK OVER THIS PROCESS OF FORMATION AND THAT EVERY FINGER AND EVERY TOE WILL DEVELOP CORRECTLY.

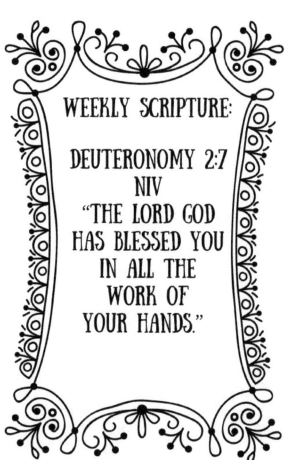

WEEKLY SCRIPTURE:

DEUTERONOMY 2:7 NIV
"THE LORD GOD HAS BLESSED YOU IN ALL THE WORK OF YOUR HANDS."

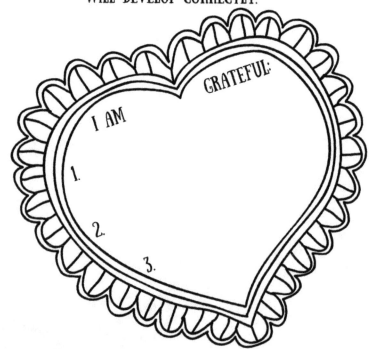

I AM GRATEFUL:

1.

2.

3.

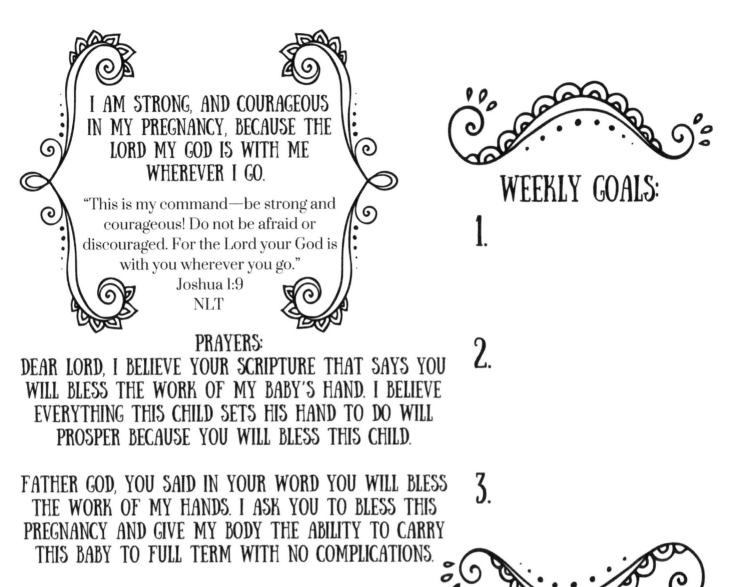

I AM STRONG, AND COURAGEOUS IN MY PREGNANCY, BECAUSE THE LORD MY GOD IS WITH ME WHEREVER I GO.

"This is my command—be strong and courageous! Do not be afraid or discouraged. For the Lord your God is with you wherever you go."
Joshua 1:9
NLT

WEEKLY GOALS:

1.

2.

3.

PRAYERS:

DEAR LORD, I BELIEVE YOUR SCRIPTURE THAT SAYS YOU WILL BLESS THE WORK OF MY BABY'S HAND. I BELIEVE EVERYTHING THIS CHILD SETS HIS HAND TO DO WILL PROSPER BECAUSE YOU WILL BLESS THIS CHILD.

FATHER GOD, YOU SAID IN YOUR WORD YOU WILL BLESS THE WORK OF MY HANDS. I ASK YOU TO BLESS THIS PREGNANCY AND GIVE MY BODY THE ABILITY TO CARRY THIS BABY TO FULL TERM WITH NO COMPLICATIONS.

THANK YOU, FATHER, FOR THE PRECIOUS FINGERS AND TOES THAT ARE GROWING AND TAKING FORM. I PRAY THEY GROW OUT PERFECTLY FROM THEIR WEBBED FORM.

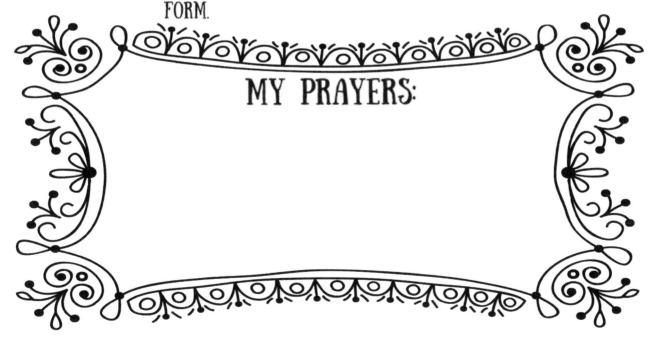

MY PRAYERS:

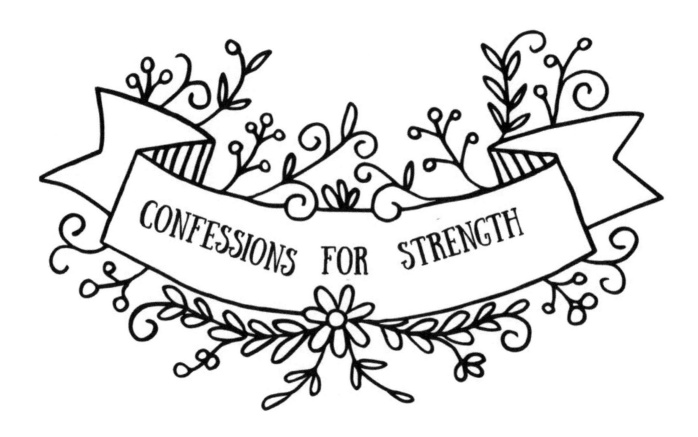

CONFESSIONS FOR STRENGTH

I am overflowing with energy and strength, as God increases my strength throughout the day!
"HE GIVES POWER TO THE TIRED AND WORN OUT, AND STRENGTH TO THE WEAK."
ISAIAH 40:29 TLB

I turn to the Lord when I am weary and worn down, and He gives me peaceful rest.
"THEN JESUS SAID, 'COME TO ME, ALL OF YOU WHO ARE WEARY AND CARRY HEAVY BURDENS, AND I WILL GIVE YOU REST.'"
MATTHEW 11:28 NLT

I am overflowing with God's strength, so I can do all things in my pregnancy.
"FOR I CAN DO EVERYTHING THROUGH CHRIST, WHO GIVES ME STRENGTH."
PHILIPPIANS 4:13 NLT

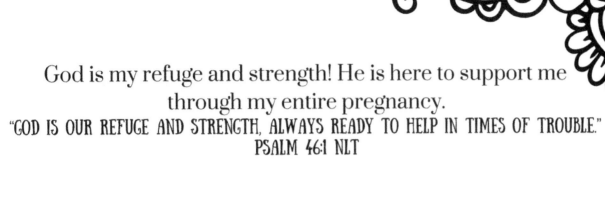

God is my refuge and strength! He is here to support me through my entire pregnancy.
"GOD IS OUR REFUGE AND STRENGTH, ALWAYS READY TO HELP IN TIMES OF TROUBLE."
PSALM 46:1 NLT

Because I love the Lord, He comes to my rescue in times of trouble. When I call on Him, He answers and gives me strength.
"THE LORD SAYS, 'I WILL RESCUE THOSE WHO LOVE ME. I WILL PROTECT THOSE WHO TRUST IN MY NAME. WHEN THEY CALL ON ME, I WILL ANSWER; I WILL BE WITH THEM IN TROUBLE. I WILL RESCUE AND HONOR THEM.'"
PSALM 91:14-15 NLT

The Lord is my light and my salvation. I have nothing to fear. I will not be afraid, because the Lord gives me strength.
"THE LORD IS MY LIGHT AND MY SALVATION; WHOM SHALL I FEAR? THE LORD IS THE STRENGTH OF MY LIFE; OF WHOM SHALL I BE AFRAID?"
PSALM 27:1 NKJV

I am strong, and courageous in my pregnancy, because the Lord my God is with me wherever I go.
"THIS IS MY COMMAND—BE STRONG AND COURAGEOUS! DO NOT BE AFRAID OR DISCOURAGED. FOR THE LORD YOUR GOD IS WITH YOU WHEREVER YOU GO."
JOSHUA 1:9 NLT

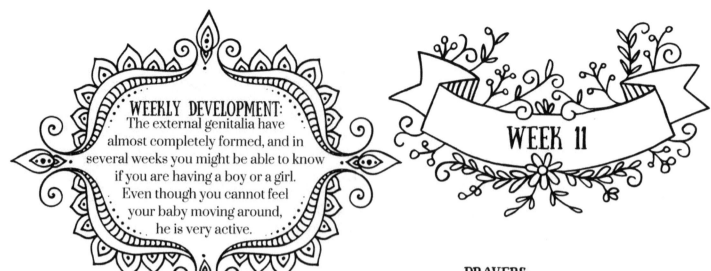

WEEK 11

WEEKLY DEVELOPMENT:
The external genitalia have almost completely formed, and in several weeks you might be able to know if you are having a boy or a girl. Even though you cannot feel your baby moving around, he is very active.

PRAYERS:
THANK YOU, LORD, THAT YOU CREATED MY BABY IN YOUR IMAGE. I KNOW THIS WEEK MY BABY'S LITTLE BOY OR LITTLE GIRL PARTS ARE ALMOST COMPLETELY FORMED, AND I AM SO THANKFUL THAT YOU HAVE DECIDED THE PERFECT GENDER FOR OUR CHILD.

TODAY I CONTINUE TO THANK YOU FOR THE BLESSINGS YOU HAVE GRANTED ME WITH THIS CHILD! I THANK YOU FOR THE ENERGY AND POSITIVITY I NEED TO BLESS THIS CHILD AS YOU HAVE BLESSED ME.

DEAR LORD, I PRAY OVER THIS VERY ACTIVE BABY. I PRAY THAT AS HE CONTINUES TO GROW, EVERY MINUTE DETAIL WILL FORM JUST AS IT SHOULD.

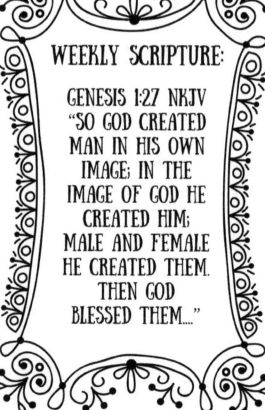

WEEKLY SCRIPTURE:

GENESIS 1:27 NKJV
"SO GOD CREATED MAN IN HIS OWN IMAGE; IN THE IMAGE OF GOD HE CREATED HIM; MALE AND FEMALE HE CREATED THEM. THEN GOD BLESSED THEM...."

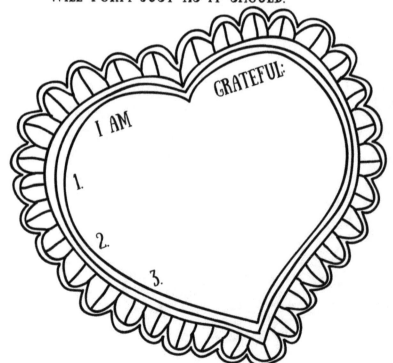

I AM GRATEFUL:

1.

2.

3.

GOD WILL NOT ALLOW ME TO SLIP AND FALL IN ANY AREA OF MY LIFE. I GIVE HIM ALL THE BURDENS OF MY PREGNANCY, AND HE TAKES CARE OF ME AND MY BABY.

"Give your burdens to the Lord, and he will take care of you. He will not permit the godly to slip and fall."
Psalm 55:22
NLT

PRAYERS:

FATHER GOD, I THANK YOU FOR YOUR PLAN FOR THIS CHILD. I THANK YOU THAT THIS BABY IS CREATED IN YOUR IMAGE, WHETHER IT IS A BOY OR A GIRL.

DEAR GOD, TODAY I ASK YOU TO PREPARE MY HEART FOR THIS SWEET CHILD. PREPARING FOR A BABY CAN BE A DAUNTING TASK, AND I ASK YOU TO GIVE ME THE WISDOM AND STRENGTH TO GET EVERYTHING COMPLETED.

HEAVENLY FATHER, I PRAY OVER MY BABY'S DADDY. I ASK YOU TO GIVE HIM PEACE AS HE IS GEARING UP TO BE A NEW DAD. GIVE HIM THE ENDURANCE TO COMFORT ME AS OUR BABY DEVELOPS.

WEEKLY GOALS:

1.

2.

3.

MY PRAYERS:

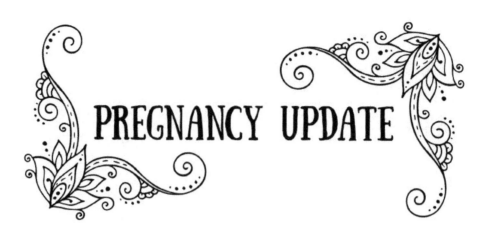

PREGNANCY UPDATE

EMOTIONS I'M FEELING:

_____
_____
_____
_____

PREGNANCY SYMPTOMS:

_____
_____
_____
_____

FOODS:

CAN'T GET ENOUGH:

_____
_____
_____

CAN'T STAND:

_____
_____

FAVORITE PREGNANCY OUTFIT:

_____
_____
_____
_____

NOTES TO MY BABY:

_____
_____
_____
_____

BABY OR BUMP
PICTURE

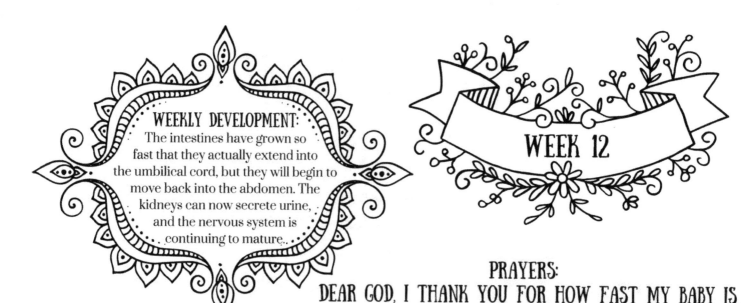

WEEKLY DEVELOPMENT:
The intestines have grown so fast that they actually extend into the umbilical cord, but they will begin to move back into the abdomen. The kidneys can now secrete urine, and the nervous system is continuing to mature.

WEEK 12

PRAYERS:

DEAR GOD, I THANK YOU FOR HOW FAST MY BABY IS GROWING. I PRAY OVER ALL OF THE INTESTINES AND THAT YOU WILL MAKE EVERY SINGLE PIECE OF THEM FORM CORRECTLY.

DEAR HEAVENLY FATHER, THANK YOU FOR CREATING MY CHILD'S INMOST BEING. I ASK YOU TO HELP THE INTESTINES TO CONTINUE TO GROW ACCORDING TO YOUR PERFECT PLAN.

LORD GOD, TODAY I PRAY FOR MY BABY'S KIDNEYS. I SPEAK OVER BOTH KIDNEYS THAT THEY WILL FORM CORRECTLY AND NEVER RUN INTO ANY PROBLEMS DURING THE LIFE OF THIS CHILD.

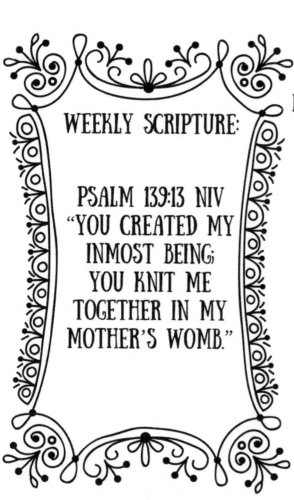

WEEKLY SCRIPTURE:

PSALM 139:13 NIV
"YOU CREATED MY INMOST BEING; YOU KNIT ME TOGETHER IN MY MOTHER'S WOMB."

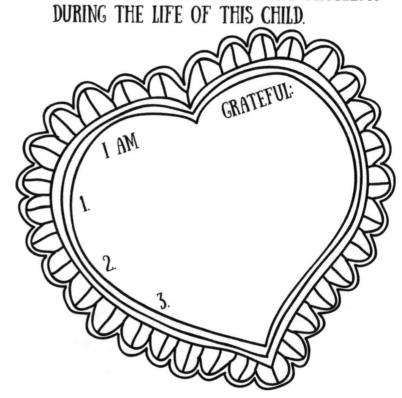

I AM GRATEFUL:

1.

2.

3.

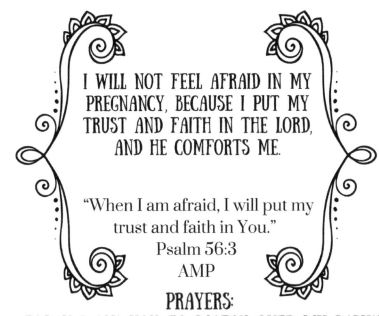

I WILL NOT FEEL AFRAID IN MY PREGNANCY, BECAUSE I PUT MY TRUST AND FAITH IN THE LORD, AND HE COMFORTS ME.

"When I am afraid, I will put my trust and faith in You."
Psalm 56:3
AMP

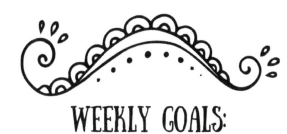

WEEKLY GOALS:

1.

2.

3.

PRAYERS:

TODAY I ASK YOU TO WATCH OVER MY BABY'S NERVOUS SYSTEM AND ENSURE THAT EVERY MINUTE DETAIL FORMS EXACTLY AS IT SHOULD IN THIS COMPLICATED SYSTEM.

DEAR LORD, I PRAY OVER THIS CHILD'S SPINAL CORD. I PRAY IT WILL GROW STRAIGHT AND THAT EVERY NERVE IN THE SPINAL CORD WILL DEVELOP FLAWLESSLY TO ALLOW THE WHOLE BODY TO FUNCTION EFFORTLESSLY.

FATHER GOD, I THANK YOU THAT YOU KNIT MY BABY TOGETHER IN MY WOMB PIECE BY PIECE. I CONTINUE TO PRAY OVER ALL THE ORGANS THAT ARE DEVELOPING THIS WEEK AND THAT THEY WILL WORK OPTIMALLY FROM THE MOMENT MY BABY IS BORN.

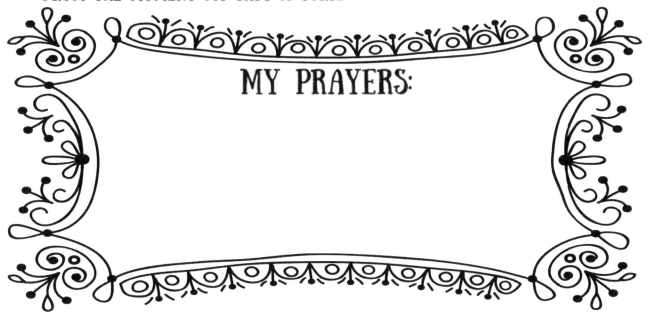

MY PRAYERS:

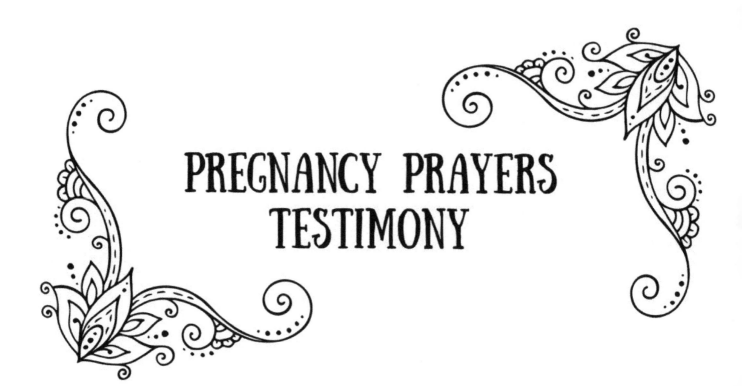

PREGNANCY PRAYERS TESTIMONY

As one can imagine, becoming a dad, especially for the first time, can be a stressful and transformational experience; one experience this dad was unprepared for. Luckily, I found the amazing Pregnancy Prayers app. Also for dads, it helps to keep track of the baby's development and brings comfort when you feel anxious. Not only do "daily prayers" inspire me to become a better individual for my kiddo, but also they cure the stress and worry that my wife and I discover.
—Robert

Download the Pregnancy Prayers app in iTunes and the Google Play stores.

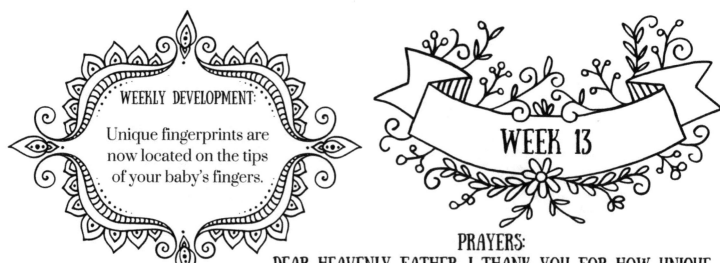

WEEKLY DEVELOPMENT:

Unique fingerprints are now located on the tips of your baby's fingers.

WEEK 13

PRAYERS:

DEAR HEAVENLY FATHER, I THANK YOU FOR HOW UNIQUE AND SPECIAL MY BABY IS. I PRAY OVER THE LITTLE FINGERS THAT NOW HAVE THEIR OWN DISTINCTIVE FINGERPRINTS.

LORD, I PRAY YOU WILL CONTINUE ON YOUR PERFECT PLAN TO FINISH YOUR MARVELOUS WORKMANSHIP IN THIS CHILD. HELP BOTH MOMMY AND DADDY WALK IN YOUR PERFECT PLAN TO ALLOW THE BEST FOR THIS BABY.

DEAR GOD, I KNOW YOU HAVE A SPECIAL PLAN FOR THIS BABY'S LIFE, AND I PRAY YOU WILL HELP HIM TO ALWAYS WALK THE PATH YOU HAVE SET UP FOR HIM. USE ME TO GUIDE HIM ALONG THE UNIQUE PATH FOR HIS LIFE.

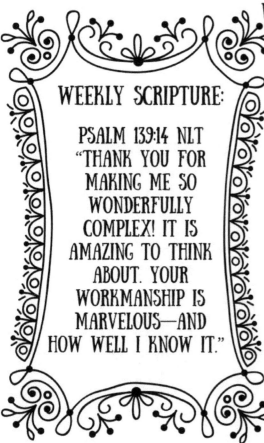

WEEKLY SCRIPTURE:

PSALM 139:14 NLT "THANK YOU FOR MAKING ME SO WONDERFULLY COMPLEX! IT IS AMAZING TO THINK ABOUT. YOUR WORKMANSHIP IS MARVELOUS—AND HOW WELL I KNOW IT."

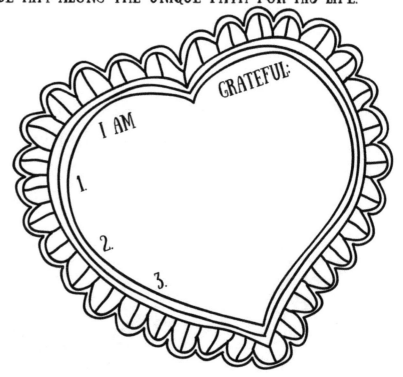

I AM GRATEFUL:

1.

2.

3.

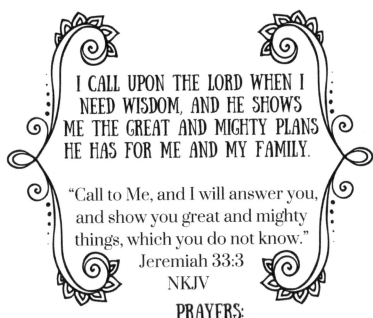

I CALL UPON THE LORD WHEN I NEED WISDOM, AND HE SHOWS ME THE GREAT AND MIGHTY PLANS HE HAS FOR ME AND MY FAMILY.

"Call to Me, and I will answer you, and show you great and mighty things, which you do not know."
Jeremiah 33:3
NKJV

WEEKLY GOALS:

1.

2.

3.

PRAYERS:

TODAY I THANK YOU FOR GIVING ME THE GRACE TO MAKE IT THROUGH THIS FIRST TRIMESTER. I SPEAK PEACE OVER THIS PREGNANCY AND ASK FOR YOUR HELP TO BRING MY CHILD DOWN THAT RIGHT PATH THROUGH THESE NEXT TWO TRIMESTERS.

HEAVENLY FATHER, I PRAY THAT YOU SEE MY HEART AND SEE HOW GRATEFUL IT IS FOR THE BLESSING OF THIS CHILD. THE WORKS OF YOUR HAND ARE TRULY MARVELOUS!

DEAR LORD, I PRAY OVER EACH FINGER AND TOE AND HOW SPECIAL THEY ARE. I AM WAITING WITH EXCITEMENT TO SEE THOSE FIRST FOOTPRINTS AND HANDPRINTS WHEN THIS SWEET BABY IS BORN.

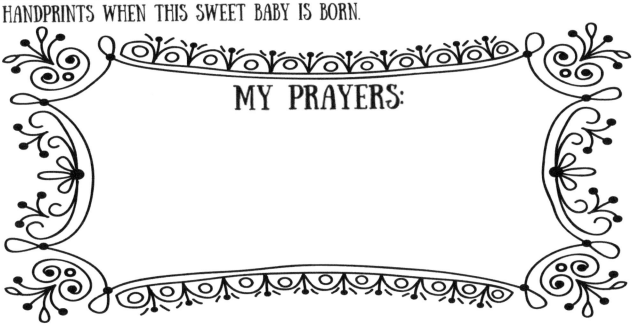

MY PRAYERS:

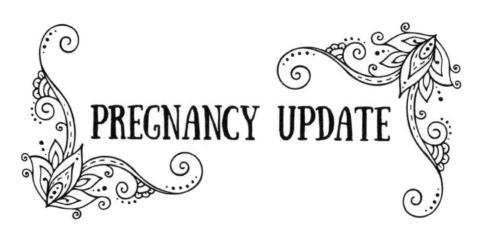

PREGNANCY UPDATE

EMOTIONS I'M FEELING:

_____
_____
_____

PREGNANCY SYMPTOMS:

_____
_____
_____
_____

FOODS:

CAN'T GET ENOUGH: CAN'T STAND:

_____   _____
_____   _____
_____

FAVORITE PREGNANCY OUTFIT:

_____
_____
_____

NOTES TO MY BABY:

_____
_____
_____
_____

BABY OR BUMP
PICTURE

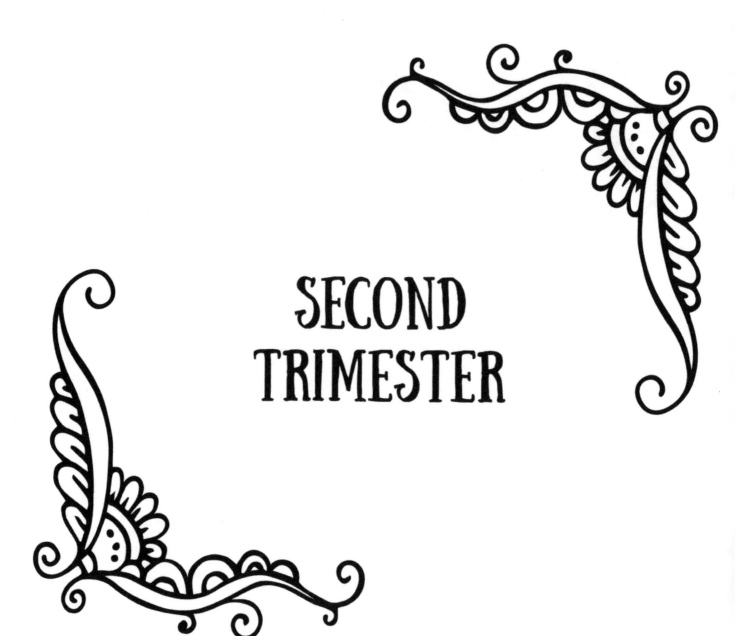

SECOND TRIMESTER

I keep my eyes
always on the LORD.
With him at my
right hand,
I will not be
shaken.
Psalm 16:8
NIV

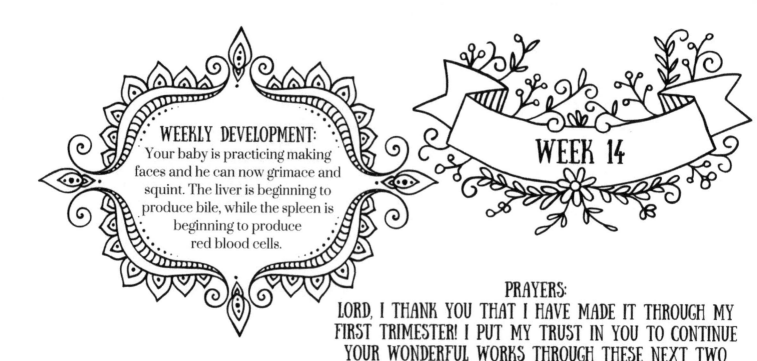

WEEKLY DEVELOPMENT:
Your baby is practicing making faces and he can now grimace and squint. The liver is beginning to produce bile, while the spleen is beginning to produce red blood cells.

WEEK 14

PRAYERS:
LORD, I THANK YOU THAT I HAVE MADE IT THROUGH MY FIRST TRIMESTER! I PUT MY TRUST IN YOU TO CONTINUE YOUR WONDERFUL WORKS THROUGH THESE NEXT TWO TRIMESTERS.

DEAR LORD, I PRAY OVER THE SWEET FACES THAT MY BABY IS MAKING. I THANK YOU THAT ALL OF THE MUSCLES HAVE FORMED PROPERLY AND WILL CONTINUE TO GROW AND STRENGTHEN AS THEY SHOULD.

TODAY I PRAY OVER MY BABY'S SPLEEN AS IT CONTINUES TO DEVELOP. I BELIEVE IT WILL FULLY DEVELOP AND FUNCTION PROPERLY IN ORDER TO PRODUCE RED BLOOD CELLS LIKE IT IS CREATED TO DO.

WEEKLY SCRIPTURE:

PHILIPPIANS 4:6-7 TLB
"DON'T WORRY ABOUT ANYTHING; INSTEAD, PRAY ABOUT EVERYTHING; TELL GOD YOUR NEEDS, AND DON'T FORGET TO THANK HIM FOR HIS ANSWERS. IF YOU DO THIS, YOU WILL EXPERIENCE GOD'S PEACE, WHICH IS FAR MORE WONDERFUL THAN THE HUMAN MIND CAN UNDERSTAND. HIS PEACE WILL KEEP YOUR THOUGHTS AND YOUR HEARTS QUIET AND AT REST AS YOU TRUST IN CHRIST JESUS."

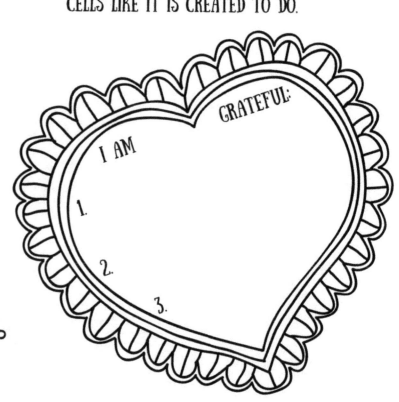

I AM GRATEFUL:
1.
2.
3.

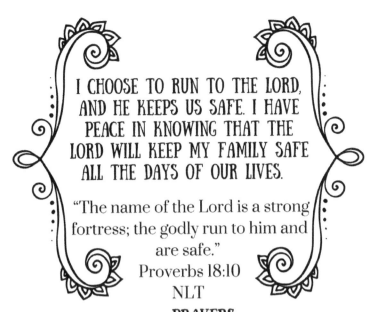

I CHOOSE TO RUN TO THE LORD, AND HE KEEPS US SAFE. I HAVE PEACE IN KNOWING THAT THE LORD WILL KEEP MY FAMILY SAFE ALL THE DAYS OF OUR LIVES.

"The name of the Lord is a strong fortress; the godly run to him and are safe."
Proverbs 18:10
NLT

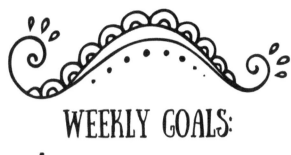

WEEKLY GOALS:

1.

2.

3.

PRAYERS:

HEAVENLY FATHER, I PRAY FOR THE CONTINUED DEVELOPMENT OF MY BABY'S LIVER. I THANK YOU THAT IT CAN ALREADY FUNCTION, AND I PRAY IT WILL ALWAYS CONTINUE TO FUNCTION WITH NO PROBLEMS.

DEAR GOD, I AM CONTINUING TO PRAY FOR MY BABY INSTEAD OF WORRYING ABOUT HIS DEVELOPMENT. I THANK YOU FOR YOUR PEACE THAT PASSES ALL UNDERSTANDING AND THAT IT WILL FOLLOW ME ALL THE DAYS OF MY PREGNANCY.

FATHER GOD, I PRAY OVER THE LIVER THAT IT WILL FUNCTION OPTIMALLY FROM DAY ONE TO PREVENT JAUNDICE. I THANK YOU THAT THE LIVER WILL BE ABLE TO FULLY BREAK DOWN ALL THAT THE BODY REQUIRES BEFORE BIRTH.

MY PRAYERS:

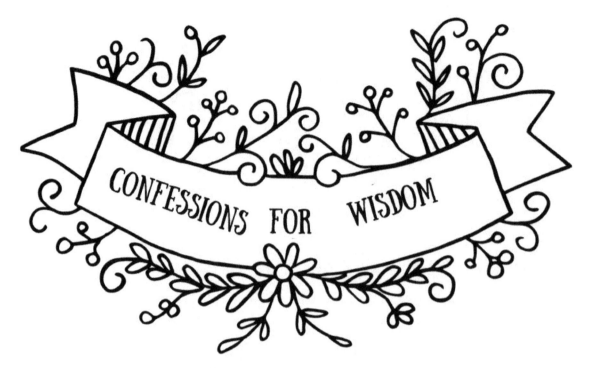

CONFESSIONS FOR WISDOM

My God will continually guide me and give me wisdom in my pregnancy. He will take care of me and my baby and satisfy us with good things.

"AND THE LORD WILL GUIDE YOU CONTINUALLY, AND SATISFY YOU WITH ALL GOOD THINGS, AND KEEP YOU HEALTHY TOO; AND YOU WILL BE LIKE A WELL-WATERED GARDEN, LIKE AN EVER-FLOWING SPRING."
ISAIAH 58:11 TLB

I am strong, and courageous in my pregnancy, because the Lord my God is with me wherever I go.

"THIS IS MY COMMAND—BE STRONG AND COURAGEOUS! DO NOT BE AFRAID OR DISCOURAGED. FOR THE LORD YOUR GOD IS WITH YOU WHEREVER YOU GO."
JOSHUA 1:9 NLT

I will seek the Lord in all I do, and He will show me which paths to take in my pregnancy.

"SEEK HIS WILL IN ALL YOU DO, AND HE WILL SHOW YOU WHICH PATH TO TAKE."
PROVERBS 3:6 NLT

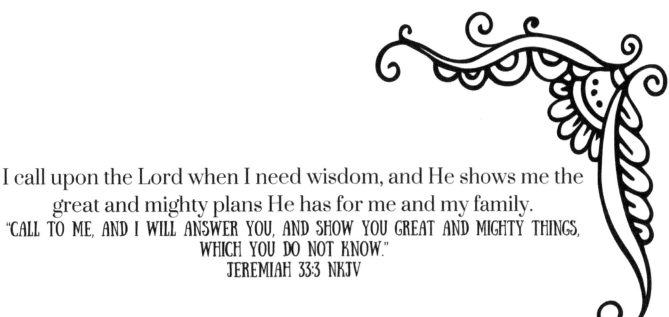

I call upon the Lord when I need wisdom, and He shows me the great and mighty plans He has for me and my family.
"CALL TO ME, AND I WILL ANSWER YOU, AND SHOW YOU GREAT AND MIGHTY THINGS, WHICH YOU DO NOT KNOW."
JEREMIAH 33:3 NKJV

God, I ask You for wisdom throughout my pregnancy, and I thank You in advance for giving it to me freely!
"IF YOU NEED WISDOM, ASK OUR GENEROUS GOD, AND HE WILL GIVE IT TO YOU. HE WILL NOT REBUKE YOU FOR ASKING."
JAMES 1:5 NLT

The Lord my God delights in every detail of my family's lives! He will direct our steps and guide us in our pregnancy.
"THE LORD DIRECTS THE STEPS OF THE GODLY. HE DELIGHTS IN EVERY DETAIL OF THEIR LIVES."
PSALM 37:23 NLT

The Lord will grant me wisdom throughout my pregnancy. I will have knowledge and understanding when it comes to caring for my baby and myself.
"FOR THE LORD GRANTS WISDOM! FROM HIS MOUTH COME KNOWLEDGE AND UNDERSTANDING."
PROVERBS 2:6 NLT

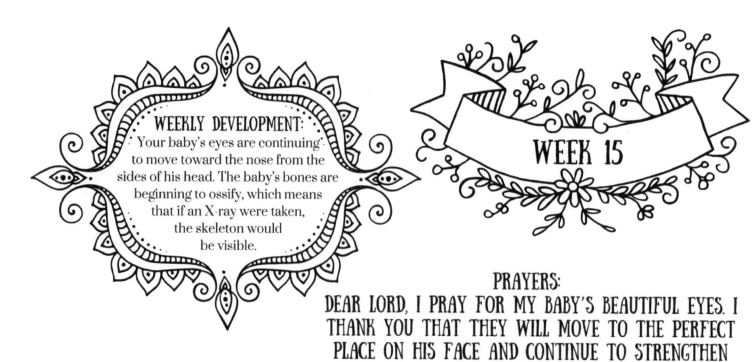

WEEKLY DEVELOPMENT:
Your baby's eyes are continuing to move toward the nose from the sides of his head. The baby's bones are beginning to ossify, which means that if an X-ray were taken, the skeleton would be visible.

WEEK 15

PRAYERS:
DEAR LORD, I PRAY FOR MY BABY'S BEAUTIFUL EYES. I THANK YOU THAT THEY WILL MOVE TO THE PERFECT PLACE ON HIS FACE AND CONTINUE TO STRENGTHEN THROUGHOUT THIS PREGNANCY.

TODAY I CONTINUE TO PRAY OVER MY BABY'S EYES, AND I PRAY THEY WILL HAVE PERFECT VISION WITH NO ABNORMALITIES. I SPEAK OVER EACH EYE AND CONFESS THAT IT WILL NEVER HAVE DISTORTIONS OR BLINDNESS.

LORD GOD, I PRAY FOR STRENGTH IN ALL OF MY BABY'S BONES. I BELIEVE THEY WILL NEVER BE WEAK OR BRITTLE, BUT THEY WILL ALWAYS HAVE YOUR STRENGTH.

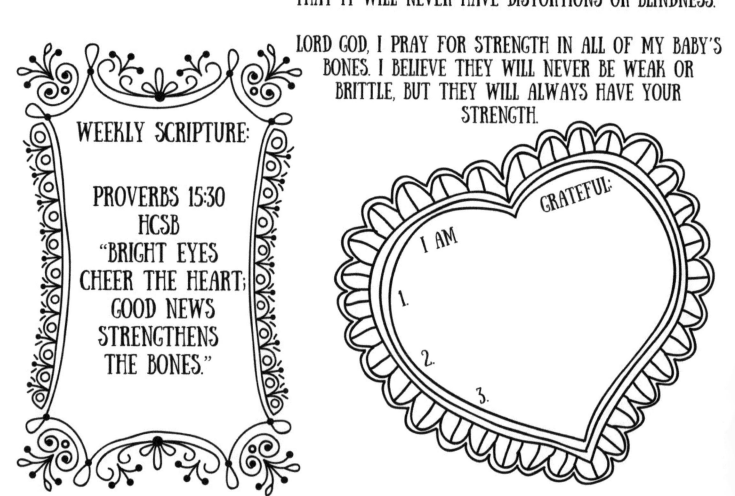

WEEKLY SCRIPTURE:

PROVERBS 15:30 HCSB
"BRIGHT EYES CHEER THE HEART; GOOD NEWS STRENGTHENS THE BONES."

I AM GRATEFUL:
1.
2.
3.

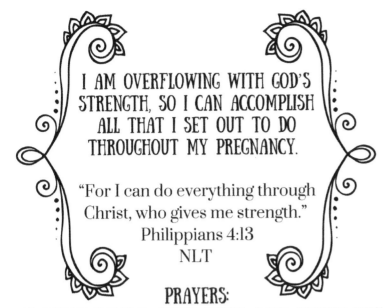

I AM OVERFLOWING WITH GOD'S STRENGTH, SO I CAN ACCOMPLISH ALL THAT I SET OUT TO DO THROUGHOUT MY PREGNANCY.

"For I can do everything through Christ, who gives me strength."
Philippians 4:13
NLT

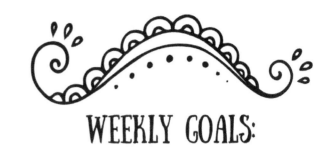

WEEKLY GOALS:

1.

2.

3.

PRAYERS:

HEAVENLY FATHER, YOUR WORD SAYS BRIGHT EYES CHEER THE HEART, AND I PRAY MY BABY WILL ALWAYS HAVE A CHEERFUL HEART. THIS HEART WILL BE BLESSED AND NEVER BITTER OR UNLOVING BUT ALWAYS FULL OF GOD'S CHEER.

DEAR GOD, I THANK YOU FOR THIS WONDERFUL BABY. I ASK YOU TO HELP ME, AND THE BABY'S DADDY, TO ALWAYS BE GOOD EXAMPLES OF A CHEERFUL HEART, AND KEEP YOUR LOVE AT THE CENTER OF OUR FAMILY.

LORD, I PRAY OVER THE OSSIFICATION PROCESS THAT IS BEGINNING IN MY BABY'S BONES. I PRAY OVER EVERY SINGLE BONE, FROM BIG TO SMALL, IN THIS LITTLE BODY. I THANK YOU THAT EACH ONE WILL GROW STRONG WITH MY BABY AS HE DEVELOPS.

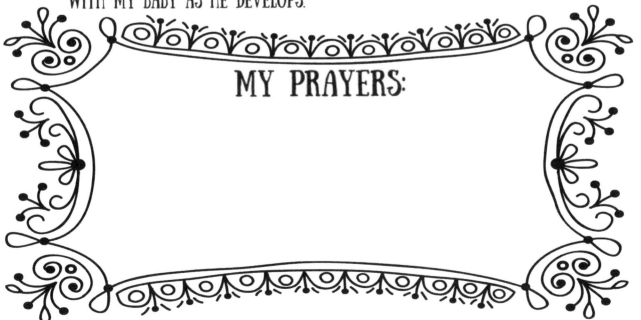

MY PRAYERS:

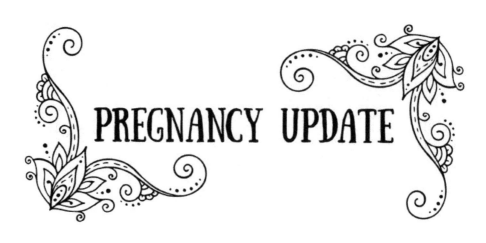

PREGNANCY UPDATE

EMOTIONS I'M FEELING:

_____
_____
_____
_____

PREGNANCY SYMPTOMS:

_____
_____
_____
_____

FOODS:

CAN'T GET ENOUGH:

_____
_____

CAN'T STAND:

_____
_____

FAVORITE PREGNANCY OUTFIT:

_____
_____
_____

NOTES TO MY BABY:

_____
_____
_____
_____

BABY OR BUMP PICTURE

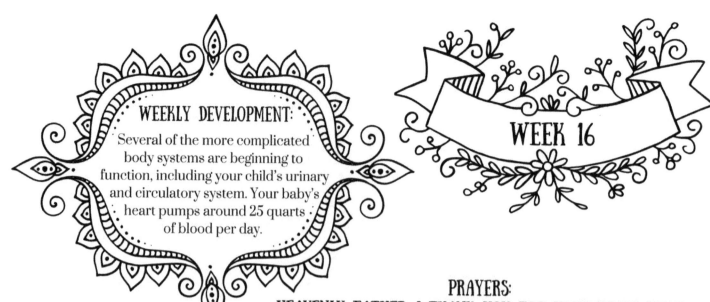

WEEKLY DEVELOPMENT:

Several of the more complicated body systems are beginning to function, including your child's urinary and circulatory system. Your baby's heart pumps around 25 quarts of blood per day.

WEEK 16

PRAYERS:

HEAVENLY FATHER, I THANK YOU FOR YOUR PEACE THAT YOUR WORD SAYS YOU WILL GIVE ME. I KNOW I WILL BE FINDING OUT THE GENDER OF OUR BABY SOON, AND I THANK YOU THAT I HAVE PEACE GOING INTO THE SONOGRAM.

TODAY I THANK YOU THAT YOU SAID OUR HEARTS SHOULD NOT BE TROUBLED OR AFRAID. I ASK YOU TO WATCH OVER THIS BABY'S HEART AND THAT IT WILL NEVER BE A TROUBLED OR FEARFUL HEART.

DEAR GOD, I BELIEVE THIS BABY'S HEART IS DEVELOPING CORRECTLY. I PRAY OVER EACH VENTRICLE, AND SAY IT IS PUMPING JUST AS IT SHOULD.

WEEKLY SCRIPTURE:

JOHN 14:27 NKJV
"PEACE I LEAVE WITH YOU, MY PEACE I GIVE TO YOU; NOT AS THE WORLD GIVES DO I GIVE TO YOU. LET NOT YOUR HEART BE TROUBLED, NEITHER LET IT BE AFRAID."

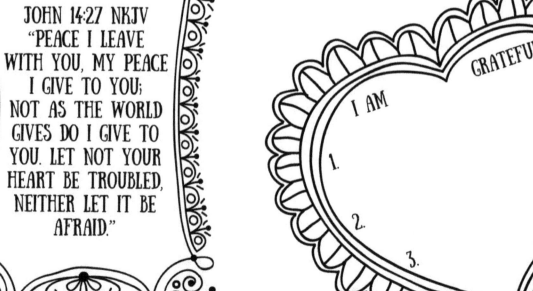

I AM GRATEFUL:

1.

2.

3.

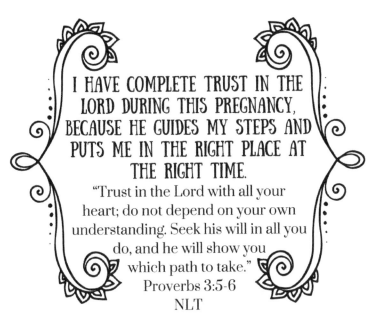

I HAVE COMPLETE TRUST IN THE LORD DURING THIS PREGNANCY, BECAUSE HE GUIDES MY STEPS AND PUTS ME IN THE RIGHT PLACE AT THE RIGHT TIME.

"Trust in the Lord with all your heart; do not depend on your own understanding. Seek his will in all you do, and he will show you which path to take."
Proverbs 3:5-6
NLT

WEEKLY GOALS:

1.

2.

3.

PRAYERS:

LORD, I PRAY FOR PEACE IN OUR FAMILY. I THANK YOU THAT YOU SAID YOU WILL LEAVE PEACE WITH US. I PRAY THERE WILL ALWAYS BE PEACE BETWEEN ME AND THIS BABY'S FATHER.

DEAR LORD, I THANK YOU THAT MY BABY'S CIRCULATORY SYSTEM IS DEVELOPING INTO THE PERFECT TRANSPORTATION CENTER FOR THIS BABY'S BODY. I ASK YOU TO CONTINUE TO WATCH OVER THIS IMPORTANT SYSTEM, AND HELP IT TO DEVELOP PERFECTLY.

FATHER GOD, I ASK YOU TO WATCH OVER THE DEVELOPING HEART IN MY BABY'S BODY AS IT PRACTICES PUMPING BLOOD. I THANK YOU THAT IT HAS ALREADY LEARNED TO PUMP 25 QUARTS A DAY, AND I BELIEVE THOSE MUSCLES WILL CONTINUE TO GROW STRONGER EACH DAY.

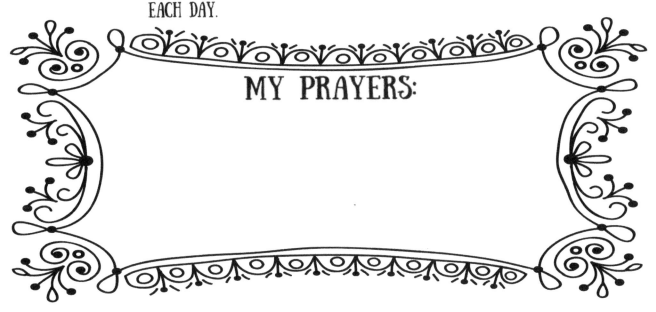

MY PRAYERS:

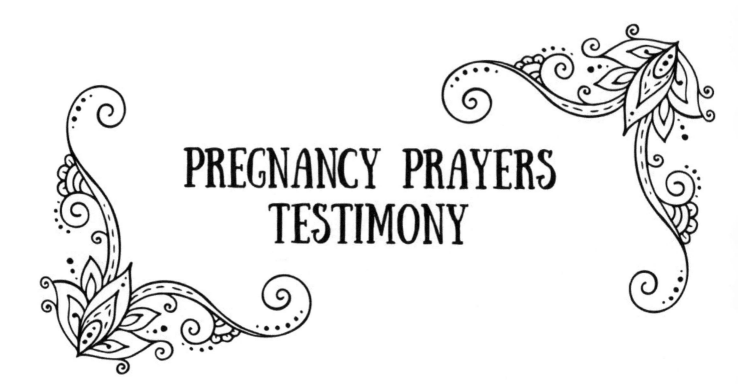

PREGNANCY PRAYERS
TESTIMONY

I am thankful for this Pregnancy Prayers app as the gift of prayer isn't my strength. I often find myself not knowing how or what to pray for. This app has helped me focus on daily prayers for my baby!

Love it!
— Leyla

Download the Pregnancy Prayers app in iTunes and the Google Play stores.

WEEKLY DEVELOPMENT:

Your baby's sense of hearing is developing since the ears have fully formed and moved into their final position.

WEEK 17

PRAYERS:

LORD, I THANK YOU FOR THE EARS THAT HAVE NOW FULLY FORMED ON MY BABY. I THANK YOU THAT EVERY PART OF THE EAR WILL FORM CORRECTLY AS THIS SWEET BABY FINISHES HIS DEVELOPMENT.

DEAR GOD, I PRAY THAT AS THESE EARS FINISH THEIR DEVELOPMENT, YOU WILL BLESS THIS BABY WITH THE ABILITY TO BE QUICK TO LISTEN AND UNDERSTAND OTHERS.

TODAY I CONTINUE TO PRAY THAT THIS BABY WILL BE QUICK TO LISTEN AND UNDERSTAND OTHERS FIRST. I PRAY OVER THE TEMPERAMENT OF THIS CHILD, AND ASK THAT HE BE SLOW TO BECOME ANGRY JUST LIKE YOUR WORD SAYS.

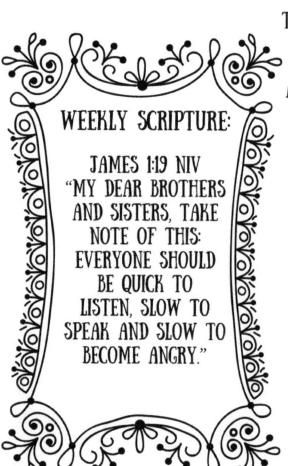

WEEKLY SCRIPTURE:

JAMES 1:19 NIV
"MY DEAR BROTHERS AND SISTERS, TAKE NOTE OF THIS: EVERYONE SHOULD BE QUICK TO LISTEN, SLOW TO SPEAK AND SLOW TO BECOME ANGRY."

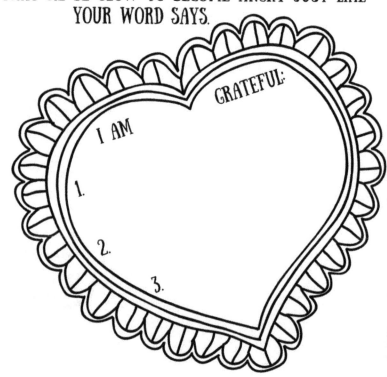

I AM GRATEFUL:

1.

2.

3.

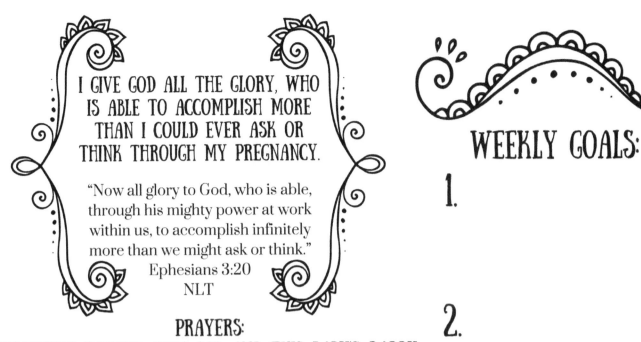

I GIVE GOD ALL THE GLORY, WHO IS ABLE TO ACCOMPLISH MORE THAN I COULD EVER ASK OR THINK THROUGH MY PREGNANCY.

"Now all glory to God, who is able, through his mighty power at work within us, to accomplish infinitely more than we might ask or think."
Ephesians 3:20
NLT

WEEKLY GOALS:

1.

2.

3.

PRAYERS:

HEAVENLY FATHER, HELP ME, AND THIS BABY'S DADDY, TO BE GOOD ROLE MODELS FOR BEING SLOW TO ANGER. SHARPEN OUR LISTENING SKILLS, AND HELP US TO SEEK UNDERSTANDING BEFORE BEING UNDERSTOOD.

FATHER GOD, I THANK YOU FOR MY BABY'S SENSE OF HEARING. I PRAY THAT ALL PARTS OF THE INNER, MIDDLE, AND OUTER EAR WILL DEVELOP TO FUNCTION OPTIMALLY FROM THE MOMENT HE IS BORN.

LORD GOD, I PRAY AGAINST EAR INFECTIONS. I KNOW HOW COMMON AND PAINFUL EAR INFECTIONS CAN BE FOR SMALL CHILDREN, AND I PRAY MY BABY WILL NOT BE PRONE TO INFECTIONS OR OTHER EAR PROBLEMS.

MY PRAYERS:

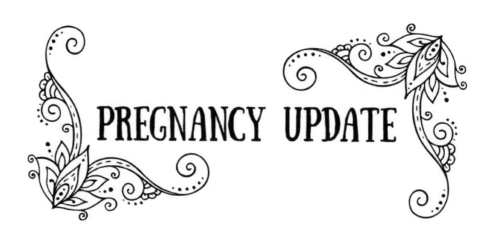

PREGNANCY UPDATE

EMOTIONS I'M FEELING:

_____
_____
_____
_____

PREGNANCY SYMPTOMS:

_____
_____
_____
_____

FOODS:

CAN'T GET ENOUGH:

_____
_____
_____

CAN'T STAND:

_____
_____

FAVORITE PREGNANCY OUTFIT:

_____
_____
_____

NOTES TO MY BABY:

_____
_____
_____
_____

BABY OR BUMP PICTURE

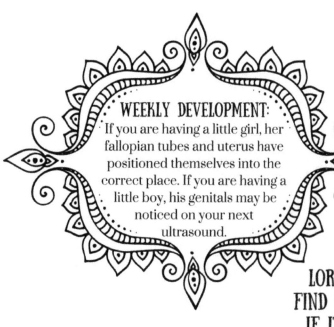

WEEKLY DEVELOPMENT:
If you are having a little girl, her fallopian tubes and uterus have positioned themselves into the correct place. If you are having a little boy, his genitals may be noticed on your next ultrasound.

WEEK 18

PRAYERS:
LORD, I ASK YOU TO PREPARE OUR HEARTS TO FIND OUT THE GENDER OF OUR SWEET BABY. EVEN IF IT IS NOT THE GENDER WE HAD PLANNED IN OUR MINDS, I ASK YOU TO GIVE US JOY IN OUR GOOD NEWS.

HEAVENLY FATHER, I THANK YOU THAT YOU HAVE A PLAN. IN A WORLD THAT FEELS SO CHAOTIC, I CHOOSE TO FIND PEACE IN YOUR PLAN TODAY.

LORD GOD, I PRAY OVER THE DEVELOPMENT OF MY BABY'S SEXUAL ORGANS. I PRAY THAT WHETHER THIS BABY IS A GIRL OR A BOY, ALL OF THE ORGANS WILL POSITION THEMSELVES IN THE CORRECT PLACE.

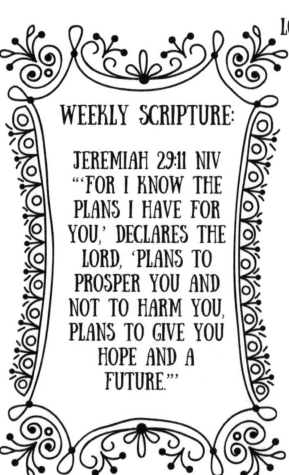

WEEKLY SCRIPTURE:

JEREMIAH 29:11 NIV
"'FOR I KNOW THE PLANS I HAVE FOR YOU,' DECLARES THE LORD, 'PLANS TO PROSPER YOU AND NOT TO HARM YOU, PLANS TO GIVE YOU HOPE AND A FUTURE.'"

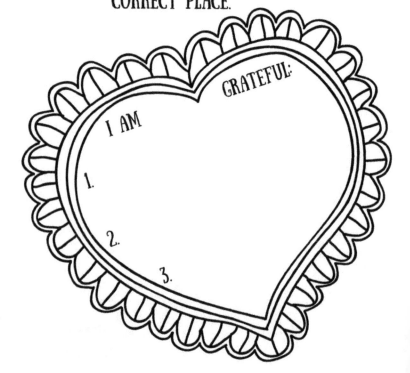

I AM GRATEFUL:

1.

2.

3.

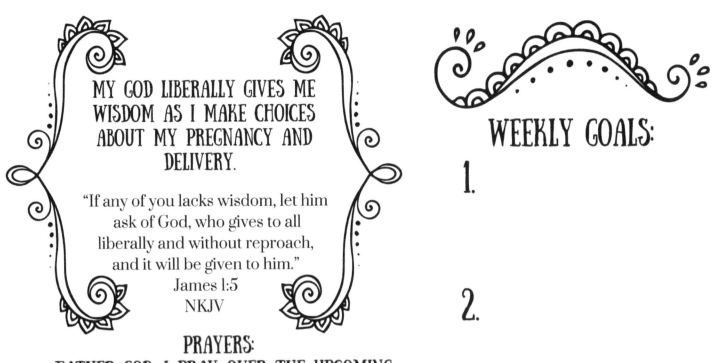

MY GOD LIBERALLY GIVES ME WISDOM AS I MAKE CHOICES ABOUT MY PREGNANCY AND DELIVERY.

"If any of you lacks wisdom, let him ask of God, who gives to all liberally and without reproach, and it will be given to him."
James 1:5
NKJV

WEEKLY GOALS:

1.

2.

3.

PRAYERS:
FATHER GOD, I PRAY OVER THE UPCOMING ULTRASOUNDS. I PRAY THAT EVERY SCAN WILL COME BACK WITH ONLY GOOD RESULTS.

HEAVENLY FATHER, I CONTINUE TO SPEAK PEACE OVER THIS PREGNANCY. I ASK FOR PEACE IN THIS FAMILY AS WE ARRANGE FOR OUR NEW BABY.

THANK YOU, FATHER, FOR GETTING US TO WEEK 18. I PRAY FOR YOUR STRENGTH AND WISDOM AS I CONTINUE IN THIS SECOND TRIMESTER.

MY PRAYERS:

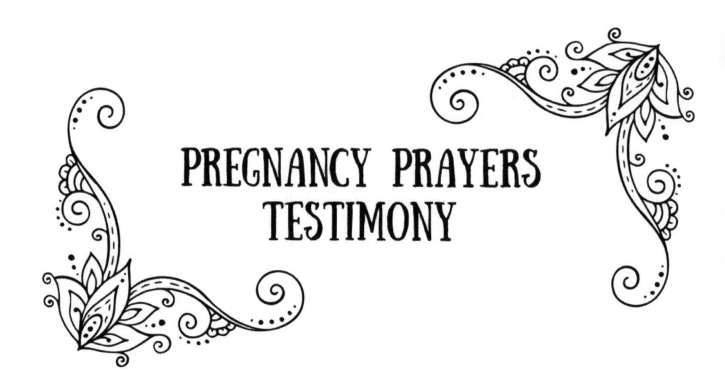

PREGNANCY PRAYERS
TESTIMONY

We have been blessed with two beautiful girls. With a third on the way we were very excited to hear we would be having a baby boy! Our family of 4 was so excited, picking names, playing dress-up with boy clothes and ready for our next adventure. One month later we were told differently. We would be having another baby girl.

I was in shock. We all were. I cried, feeing brokenhearted. We had become so attached to what we thought was our little boy. My heart could not connect to this little girl, and that too broke my heart.

On January 1, I got a Pregnancy Prayers notification. I opened it up and it read, "Lord I ask You to prepare our hearts to find out the gender of our sweet baby. Even if it is not the gender we had planned in our minds, we ask You to give us joy in our good news." Of course, I started sobbing and thanking God for this app that is a continuous reminder of how precious and present God is during this pregnancy. It was exactly what I needed to bring joy to my heart. From that moment, that became my prayer. With great joy, we can't wait to meet our third beauty!
—Aubrey

Download the Pregnancy Prayers app in iTunes and the Google Play stores.

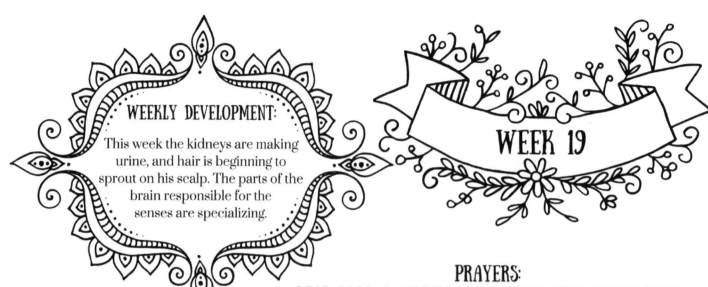

WEEKLY DEVELOPMENT:

This week the kidneys are making urine, and hair is beginning to sprout on his scalp. The parts of the brain responsible for the senses are specializing.

WEEK 19

PRAYERS:

DEAR LORD, I CONTINUE TO PRAY OVER THE KIDNEY DEVELOPMENT IN MY BABY. I PRAY HE WILL MAINTAIN HIS GROWTH, AND CARRY ON WITH HIS DEVELOPMENT UNTIL BOTH KIDNEYS ARE FULLY FUNCTIONING.

HEAVENLY FATHER, I THANK YOU FOR THE HAIR THAT IS BEGINNING TO DEVELOP ON MY BABY'S HEAD. I PRAY, EVEN THOUGH IT SEEMS INSIGNIFICANT, THAT YOU WILL GIVE MY BABY HEALTHY HAIR THROUGHOUT HIS LIFE

LORD GOD, I PRAY OVER THE INNER BEAUTY OF THIS BABY. I PRAY HE WILL HAVE A GENTLE, SWEET AND LOVING SPIRIT ALL THE DAYS OF HIS LIFE.

WEEKLY SCRIPTURE:

I PETER 3:3-4 NIV
"YOUR BEAUTY SHOULD NOT COME FROM OUTWARD ADORNMENT, SUCH AS ELABORATE HAIRSTYLES AND THE WEARING OF GOLD JEWELRY OR FINE CLOTHES. RATHER, IT SHOULD BE THAT OF YOUR INNER SELF, THE UNFADING BEAUTY OF A GENTLE AND QUIET SPIRIT, WHICH IS OF GREAT WORTH IN GOD'S SIGHT."

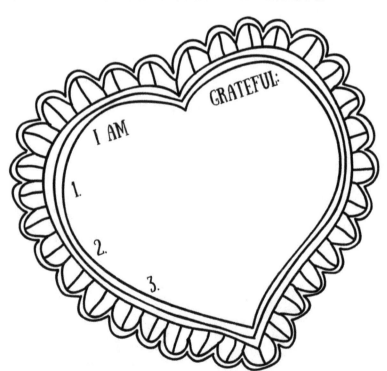

I AM GRATEFUL:

1.

2.

3.

MY BABY IS GOD'S MASTERPIECE THAT HE CREATED. HE HAS GREAT THINGS PLANNED FOR OUR FUTURE.

"For we are God's masterpiece. He has created us anew in Christ Jesus, so we can do the good things he planned for us long ago."
Ephesians 2:10
NLT

PRAYERS:
FATHER GOD, HELP OUR FAMILY TO NOT RELY ON OUTWARD BEAUTIFICATION, BUT TO ALL BE BEAUTIFUL ON THE INSIDE SO WE CAN SET A GODLY EXAMPLE FOR THIS NEW BABY.

LORD, I THANK YOU THAT THIS BABY WILL HAVE A GENTLE SPIRIT. I PRAY MY BABY WILL NOT HAVE COLIC OR ISSUES SLEEPING AS A NEWBORN, BUT THAT HE WILL BE CONTINUALLY COVERED IN YOUR PEACE.

THANK YOU, LORD, FOR THE MIRACLE OF MY BABY'S BRAIN. I PRAY OVER THE SECTIONS THAT CONTROL THE SENSES AND KEEP MY BABY ALERT TO HIS SURROUNDINGS. I THANK YOU THAT EVERY PART, NO MATTER HOW SMALL, WILL WORK TO THE FULLEST FUNCTION.

WEEKLY GOALS:

1.

2.

3.

MY PRAYERS:

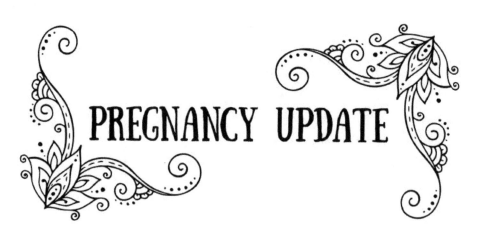

PREGNANCY UPDATE

EMOTIONS I'M FEELING:

_____
_____
_____
_____

PREGNANCY SYMPTOMS:

_____
_____
_____
_____

FOODS:

CAN'T GET ENOUGH:

_____
_____
_____

CAN'T STAND:

_____
_____
_____

FAVORITE PREGNANCY OUTFIT:

_____
_____
_____

NOTES TO MY BABY:

_____
_____
_____
_____

BABY OR BUMP
PICTURE

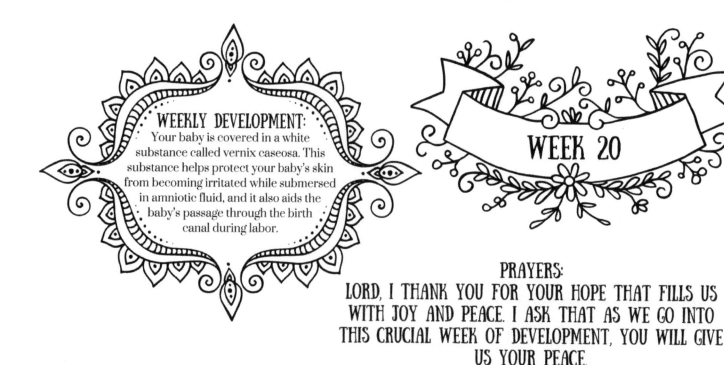

WEEKLY DEVELOPMENT:
Your baby is covered in a white substance called vernix caseosa. This substance helps protect your baby's skin from becoming irritated while submersed in amniotic fluid, and it also aids the baby's passage through the birth canal during labor.

WEEK 20

PRAYERS:
LORD, I THANK YOU FOR YOUR HOPE THAT FILLS US WITH JOY AND PEACE. I ASK THAT AS WE GO INTO THIS CRUCIAL WEEK OF DEVELOPMENT, YOU WILL GIVE US YOUR PEACE.

FATHER GOD, I PRAY OVER ULTRASOUNDS THAT HAVE BEEN TAKEN, AND WILL BE TAKEN OF THIS BABY. I PRAY THAT EACH SCAN WILL SHOW GROWTH AND DEVELOPMENT, WITHOUT ANY FORM OF ABNORMALITY.

LORD GOD, I PRAY OVER THE PROTECTIVE LAYER THAT IS COVERING MY BABY. I PRAY IT WILL WHOLLY SERVE ITS PURPOSE IN KEEPING MY BABY'S SKIN FROM BEING IRRITATED IN THE WOMB.

WEEKLY SCRIPTURE:

ROMANS 15:13 AMPC
"MAY THE GOD OF YOUR HOPE SO FILL YOU WITH ALL JOY AND PEACE IN BELIEVING [THROUGH THE EXPERIENCE OF YOUR FAITH] THAT BY THE POWER OF THE HOLY SPIRIT YOU MAY ABOUND AND BE OVERFLOWING (BUBBLING OVER) WITH HOPE."

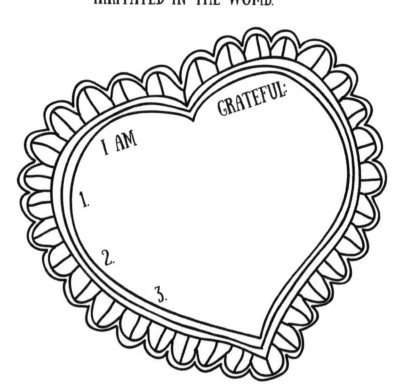

I AM GRATEFUL:
1.
2.
3.

I WILL NOT BE AFRAID OR DISCOURAGED IN MY PREGNANCY, BECAUSE MY GOD GIVES ME STRENGTH AND WILL HOLD ME UP VICTORIOUSLY.

"Don't be afraid, for I am with you. Don't be discouraged, for I am your God. I will strengthen you and help you. I will hold you up with my victorious right hand."

Isaiah 41:10
NLT

PRAYERS:

TODAY I THANK YOU FOR THE DEVELOPMENT THAT HAS TAKEN PLACE IN THIS BABY SO FAR. I THANK YOU THAT I HAVE BEEN ABLE TO CARRY THIS BABY TO THE HALF-WAY POINT, AND ASK FOR YOUR STRENGTH AS I START THE SECOND HALF OF THIS PREGNANCY.

GRACIOUS GOD, I PRAY FOR PEACE AS WE POSSIBLY SEE DETAILED SONOGRAMS OF OUR BABY. I ASK THAT IF WE HAVE CHALLENGING FINDINGS, YOU WILL CONTINUE TO GIVE US PEACE AS WE TRUST IN YOU.

HEAVENLY FATHER, I THANK YOU FOR YOUR JOY IN THIS PROCESS. I THANK YOU, EVEN IF IT DOESN'T FEEL LIKE IT, THAT TODAY WE WILL BE BUBBLING OVER WITH HOPE FOR THE FUTURE OF THIS CHILD.

WEEKLY GOALS:

1.

2.

3.

MY PRAYERS:

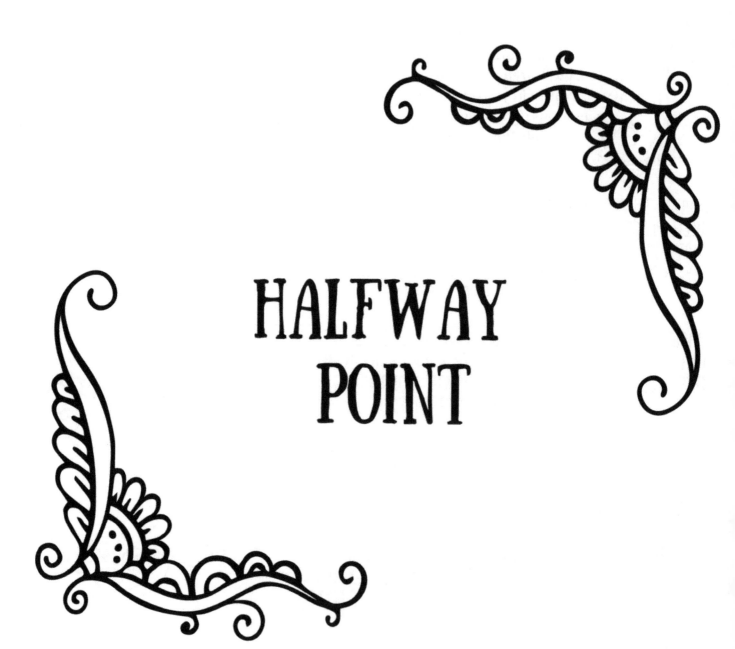

HALFWAY POINT

And I am certain that God, who began the good work within you, will continue his work until it is finally finished on the day when Christ Jesus returns.
Philippians 1:6
NLT

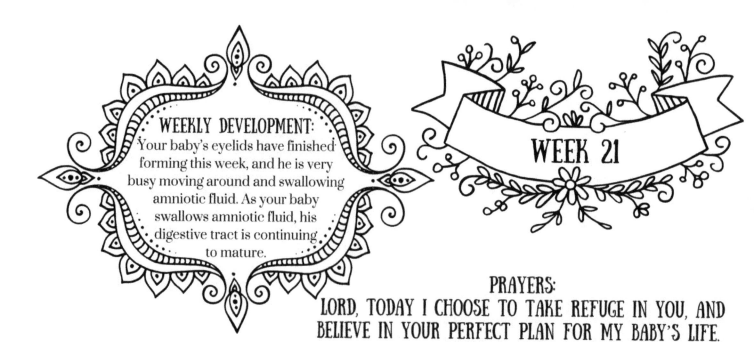

WEEKLY DEVELOPMENT: Your baby's eyelids have finished forming this week, and he is very busy moving around and swallowing amniotic fluid. As your baby swallows amniotic fluid, his digestive tract is continuing to mature.

WEEK 21

PRAYERS:

LORD, TODAY I CHOOSE TO TAKE REFUGE IN YOU, AND BELIEVE IN YOUR PERFECT PLAN FOR MY BABY'S LIFE.

FATHER GOD, I PRAY OVER THE EYELIDS THAT ARE FINISHED FORMING THIS WEEK. I PRAY THAT BOTH EYELIDS WILL HAVE FORMED JUST AS THEY SHOULD TO PROTECT MY BABY'S EYES.

THANK YOU FOR MY HEALTHY, ACTIVE BABY! I THANK YOU THAT WE HAVE MADE IT ANOTHER WEEK IN THIS PREGNANCY. I CHOOSE TO BELIEVE THAT NO MATTER HOW I AM FEELING, OR HOW CIRCUMSTANCES APPEAR, THE LORD IS GOOD.

WEEKLY SCRIPTURE:

PSALM 34:8 HCSB
"TASTE AND SEE THAT THE LORD IS GOOD.
HOW HAPPY IS THE MAN WHO TAKES REFUGE IN HIM."

I AM GRATEFUL:
1.
2.
3.

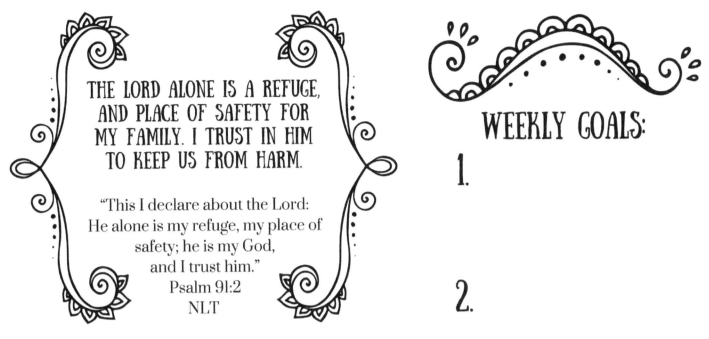

THE LORD ALONE IS A REFUGE, AND PLACE OF SAFETY FOR MY FAMILY. I TRUST IN HIM TO KEEP US FROM HARM.

"This I declare about the Lord: He alone is my refuge, my place of safety; he is my God, and I trust him."
Psalm 91:2
NLT

WEEKLY GOALS:

1.

2.

3.

PRAYERS:

GRACIOUS GOD, I PRAY OVER THIS BABY'S DIGESTIVE TRACT. I PRAY AS IT PRACTICES PROCESSING AMNIOTIC FLUID, IT WILL LEARN TO FUNCTION ENTIRELY.

LORD GOD, I PRAY OVER MY UPCOMING LABOR, EVEN THOUGH IT'S STILL SEVERAL WEEKS OUT. I PRAY THAT IT WILL BE A SMOOTH AND EASY PROCESS.

HEAVENLY FATHER, HELP OUR FAMILY WORK TOGETHER TO SHOW THIS BABY HOW TO TAKE REFUGE IN YOU, AND BE HAPPY. I PRAY THIS BABY WILL KNOW PURE HAPPINESS, AND BE A JOYFUL BABY.

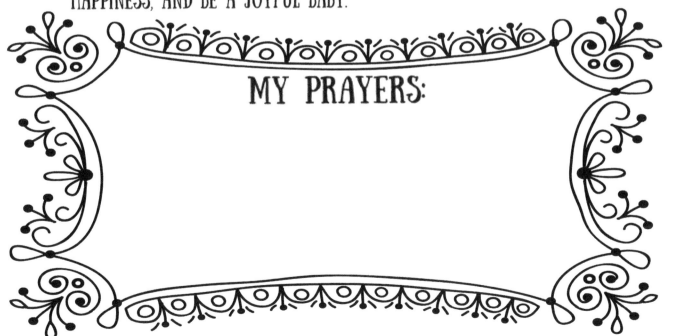

MY PRAYERS:

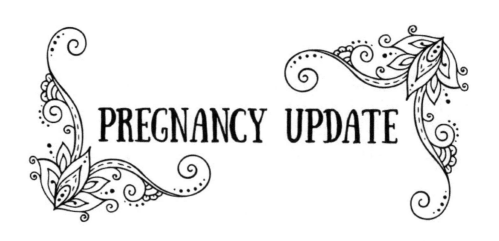

PREGNANCY UPDATE

EMOTIONS I'M FEELING:

_____
_____
_____

PREGNANCY SYMPTOMS:

_____
_____
_____

FOODS:

CAN'T GET ENOUGH:

_____
_____
_____

CAN'T STAND:

_____
_____

FAVORITE PREGNANCY OUTFIT:

_____
_____
_____

NOTES TO MY BABY:

_____
_____
_____
_____

BABY OR BUMP PICTURE

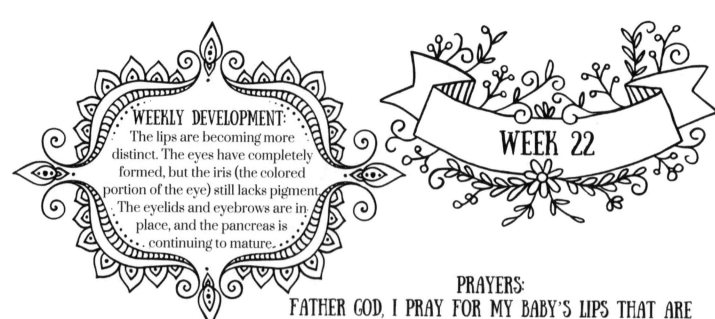

WEEKLY DEVELOPMENT:
The lips are becoming more distinct. The eyes have completely formed, but the iris (the colored portion of the eye) still lacks pigment. The eyelids and eyebrows are in place, and the pancreas is continuing to mature.

WEEK 22

PRAYERS:
FATHER GOD, I PRAY FOR MY BABY'S LIPS THAT ARE FILLING OUT AND BECOMING DISTINCT. I PRAY THIS BABY'S LIPS WILL GLORIFY YOU ALL THE DAYS OF HIS LIFE.

LORD, HELP MY LIPS TO ALWAYS GLORIFY YOU, SO I CAN SET THE EXAMPLE FOR MY BABY. HELP ME SPEAK ONLY POSITIVE WORDS OVER MY BODY AND THIS CHILD.

HEAVENLY FATHER, I THANK YOU THAT MY BABY'S EYES ARE COMPLETELY FORMED. I PRAY THEY HAVE FORMED CORRECTLY, AND THE IRIS WILL FINISH ITS DEVELOPMENT AND GAIN THE PERFECT COLOR PIGMENT.

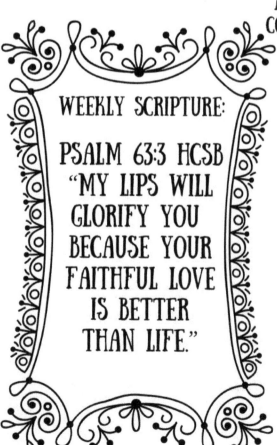

WEEKLY SCRIPTURE:

PSALM 63:3 HCSB
"MY LIPS WILL GLORIFY YOU BECAUSE YOUR FAITHFUL LOVE IS BETTER THAN LIFE."

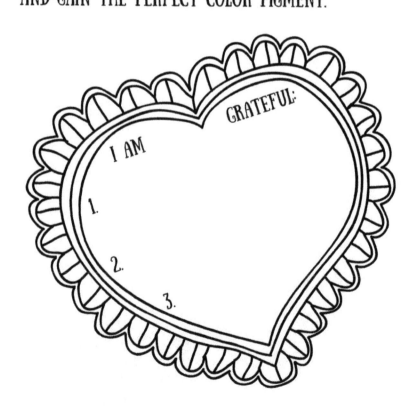

I AM   GRATEFUL:

1.

2.

3.

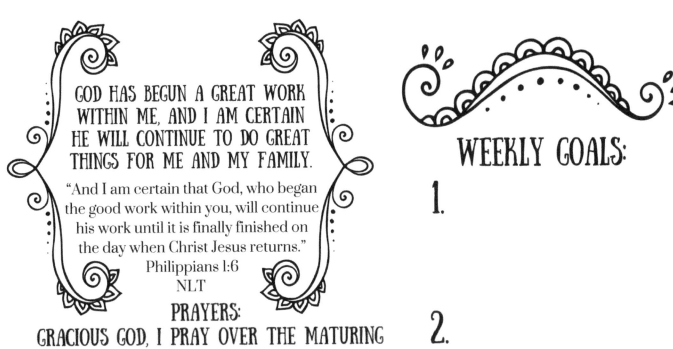

GOD HAS BEGUN A GREAT WORK WITHIN ME, AND I AM CERTAIN HE WILL CONTINUE TO DO GREAT THINGS FOR ME AND MY FAMILY.

"And I am certain that God, who began the good work within you, will continue his work until it is finally finished on the day when Christ Jesus returns."
Philippians 1:6
NLT

WEEKLY GOALS:

1.

2.

3.

PRAYERS:

GRACIOUS GOD, I PRAY OVER THE MATURING PANCREAS. I PRAY IT WILL NATURALLY PRODUCE THE DIGESTIVE JUICES AND INSULIN THAT IT WAS CREATED TO GENERATE.

LORD GOD, I PRAY THAT AS LABOR AND DELIVERY DRAW CLOSER, I WILL NOT BE ANXIOUS. I THANK YOU THAT YOU HAVE A PERFECT DAY PLANNED FOR MY DELIVERY, AND I WILL HAVE A SENSE OF CALM THROUGHOUT THE PROCESS.

TODAY I THANK YOU FOR MY BABY'S EYES. I THANK YOU THAT YOUR WORD SAYS OUR EYES ARE BLESSED TO SEE, AND THIS BABY WILL ALWAYS HAVE THE BLESSING OF SIGHT!

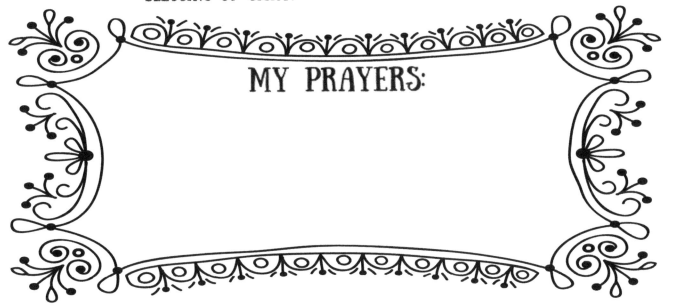

MY PRAYERS:

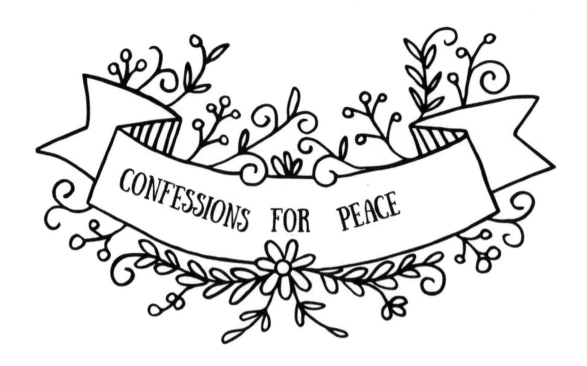

CONFESSIONS FOR PEACE

I am completely filled with joy and peace about my pregnancy and my baby, because I am overflowing with God's confident hope!

"I PRAY THAT GOD, THE SOURCE OF HOPE, WILL FILL YOU COMPLETELY WITH JOY AND PEACE BECAUSE YOU TRUST IN HIM. THEN YOU WILL OVERFLOW WITH CONFIDENT HOPE THROUGH THE POWER OF THE HOLY SPIRIT."
ROMANS 15:13 NLT

I will not be afraid or discouraged about my family's future. My God will strengthen us and hold us victoriously in His right hand. He will never leave us or forsake us!

"DON'T BE AFRAID, FOR I AM WITH YOU. DON'T BE DISCOURAGED, FOR I AM YOUR GOD. I WILL STRENGTHEN YOU AND HELP YOU. I WILL HOLD YOU UP WITH MY VICTORIOUS RIGHT HAND."
ISAIAH 41:10 NLT

I will not be shaken during my pregnancy, because God is my rock and salvation.

"HE ALONE IS MY ROCK AND MY SALVATION, MY FORTRESS WHERE I WILL NOT BE SHAKEN."
PSALM 62:6 NLT

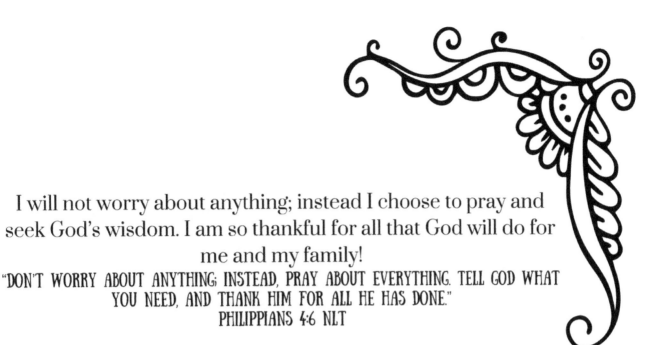

I will not worry about anything; instead I choose to pray and seek God's wisdom. I am so thankful for all that God will do for me and my family!

"DON'T WORRY ABOUT ANYTHING; INSTEAD, PRAY ABOUT EVERYTHING. TELL GOD WHAT YOU NEED, AND THANK HIM FOR ALL HE HAS DONE."
PHILIPPIANS 4:6 NLT

I give all my worries and all my cares to God! He loves me and my baby, and He takes care of us.

"GIVE ALL YOUR WORRIES AND CARES TO GOD, FOR HE CARES ABOUT YOU."
1 PETER 5:7 NLT

I will enjoy great peace in my pregnancy, because I am a child of God. My home and family will overflow with the love of God and His peace.

"I WILL TEACH ALL YOUR CHILDREN, AND THEY WILL ENJOY GREAT PEACE."
ISAIAH 54:13 NLT

My God gives me peace at all times and in all situations. I choose to accept His peace no matter what circumstances I face.

"NOW MAY THE LORD OF PEACE HIMSELF GIVE YOU HIS PEACE AT ALL TIMES AND IN EVERY SITUATION. THE LORD BE WITH YOU ALL."
2 THESSALONIANS 3:16 NLT

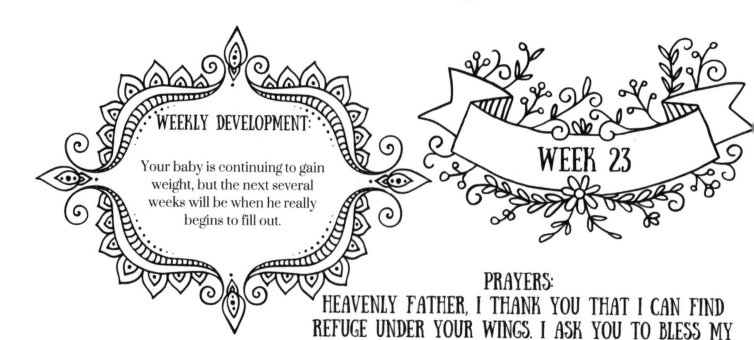

WEEKLY DEVELOPMENT:

Your baby is continuing to gain weight, but the next several weeks will be when he really begins to fill out.

WEEK 23

PRAYERS:

HEAVENLY FATHER, I THANK YOU THAT I CAN FIND REFUGE UNDER YOUR WINGS. I ASK YOU TO BLESS MY FAMILY WITH YOUR JOY AND STRENGTH AS WE GET CLOSER TO MEETING THIS NEW BABY.

LORD GOD, AS THIS BABY AND I CONTINUE TO GROW, I PRAY YOU WILL GIVE ME THE STRENGTH TO CARRY HIM TO FULL TERM. I ASK YOU TO HELP ME MANAGE PAIN AND FATIGUE THAT CAN COME WITH PREGNANCY.

THANK YOU, LORD, THAT MY BABY IS GAINING WEIGHT! I PRAY HE WILL FILL OUT TO THE PERFECT WEIGHT YOU HAVE PLANNED FOR DELIVERY.

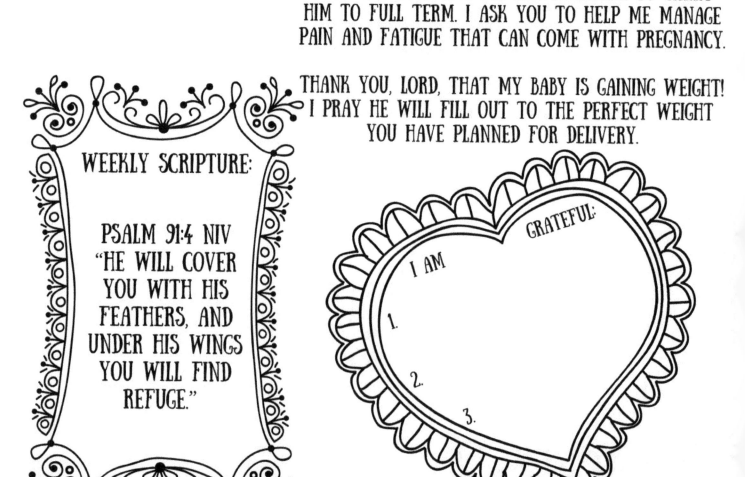

WEEKLY SCRIPTURE:

PSALM 91:4 NIV
"HE WILL COVER YOU WITH HIS FEATHERS, AND UNDER HIS WINGS YOU WILL FIND REFUGE."

I AM GRATEFUL:

1.

2.

3.

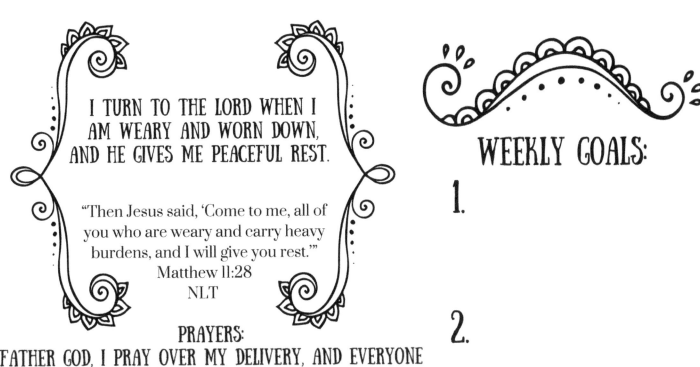

I TURN TO THE LORD WHEN I AM WEARY AND WORN DOWN, AND HE GIVES ME PEACEFUL REST.

"Then Jesus said, 'Come to me, all of you who are weary and carry heavy burdens, and I will give you rest.'"
Matthew 11:28
NLT

WEEKLY GOALS:

1.

2.

3.

PRAYERS:

FATHER GOD, I PRAY OVER MY DELIVERY, AND EVERYONE WHO WILL BE INVOLVED. I PRAY THE DOCTORS, NURSES, MIDWIVES, ETC., WILL HAVE THE WISDOM TO MAKE CRUCIAL DECISIONS TO KEEP ME AND MY BABY HEALTHY DURING DELIVERY.

GRACIOUS GOD, TAKE THIS BABY UNDER YOUR WINGS. I KNOW YOU HAVE A PLAN FOR HIS LIFE, AND I PRAY THIS BABY WILL ALWAYS BE ABLE TO FIND REFUGE IN YOU.

LORD, I PRAY OVER WEIGHT GAIN WITH THIS CHILD. I PRAY YOU WILL GIVE ME WISDOM ABOUT WHAT FOODS TO EAT NOW, AND TO FEED MY GROWING CHILD. I PRAY THIS CHILD WILL NOT HAVE TO STRUGGLE TO STAY AT A HEALTHY WEIGHT AT ANY POINT IN HIS LIFE.

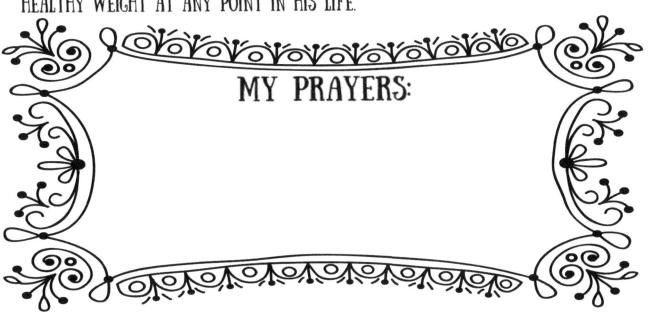

MY PRAYERS:

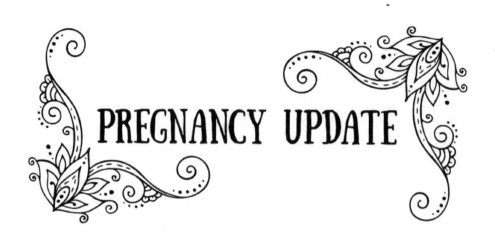

PREGNANCY UPDATE

EMOTIONS I'M FEELING:

_____
_____
_____
_____

PREGNANCY SYMPTOMS:

_____
_____
_____
_____

FOODS:

CAN'T GET ENOUGH:

_____
_____
_____

CAN'T STAND:

_____
_____

FAVORITE PREGNANCY OUTFIT:

_____
_____
_____
_____

NOTES TO MY BABY:

_____
_____
_____
_____

BABY OR BUMP PICTURE

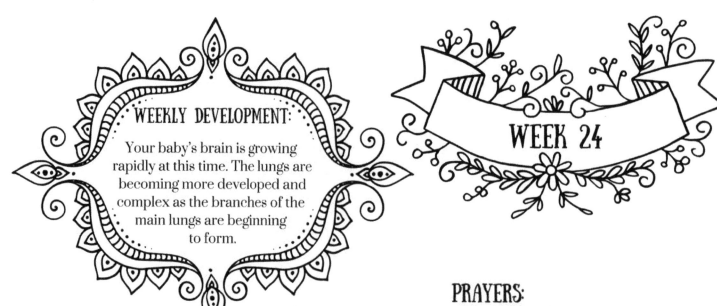

WEEKLY DEVELOPMENT:

Your baby's brain is growing rapidly at this time. The lungs are becoming more developed and complex as the branches of the main lungs are beginning to form.

WEEK 24

PRAYERS:

THANK YOU, LORD, FOR YOUR WISDOM! I ASK FOR YOUR WISDOM AS OUR FAMILY ARRANGES OUR LIVES TO ACCOMMODATE THIS SWEET BABY.

LORD GOD, I PRAY THAT AS MY BABY'S BRAIN GROWS, IT WILL BE FORMED PERFECTLY BY YOUR HANDS.

FATHER GOD, I PRAY YOU WILL BREATHE YOUR WISDOM INTO THIS BABY, SO THAT HE CAN UNDERSTAND YOU, AND GROW ACCORDING TO YOUR PERFECT PLAN.

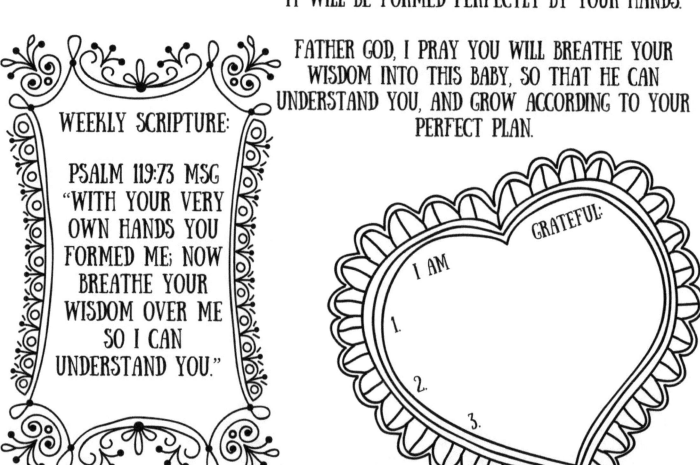

WEEKLY SCRIPTURE:

PSALM 119:73 MSG "WITH YOUR VERY OWN HANDS YOU FORMED ME; NOW BREATHE YOUR WISDOM OVER ME SO I CAN UNDERSTAND YOU."

I AM   GRATEFUL:

1.

2.

3.

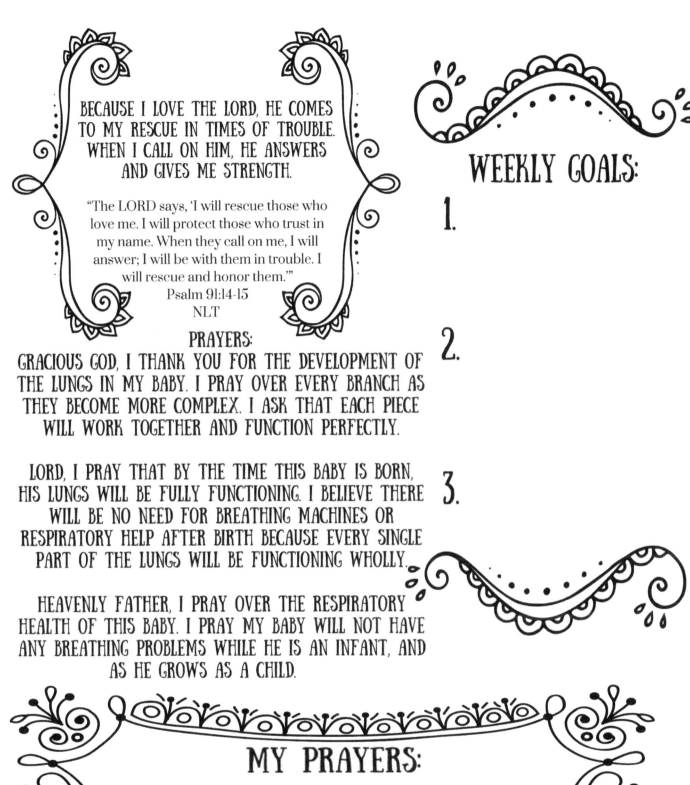

BECAUSE I LOVE THE LORD, HE COMES TO MY RESCUE IN TIMES OF TROUBLE. WHEN I CALL ON HIM, HE ANSWERS AND GIVES ME STRENGTH.

"The LORD says, 'I will rescue those who love me. I will protect those who trust in my name. When they call on me, I will answer; I will be with them in trouble. I will rescue and honor them.'"

Psalm 91:14-15
NLT

PRAYERS:

GRACIOUS GOD, I THANK YOU FOR THE DEVELOPMENT OF THE LUNGS IN MY BABY. I PRAY OVER EVERY BRANCH AS THEY BECOME MORE COMPLEX. I ASK THAT EACH PIECE WILL WORK TOGETHER AND FUNCTION PERFECTLY.

LORD, I PRAY THAT BY THE TIME THIS BABY IS BORN, HIS LUNGS WILL BE FULLY FUNCTIONING. I BELIEVE THERE WILL BE NO NEED FOR BREATHING MACHINES OR RESPIRATORY HELP AFTER BIRTH BECAUSE EVERY SINGLE PART OF THE LUNGS WILL BE FUNCTIONING WHOLLY.

HEAVENLY FATHER, I PRAY OVER THE RESPIRATORY HEALTH OF THIS BABY. I PRAY MY BABY WILL NOT HAVE ANY BREATHING PROBLEMS WHILE HE IS AN INFANT, AND AS HE GROWS AS A CHILD.

WEEKLY GOALS:

1.

2.

3.

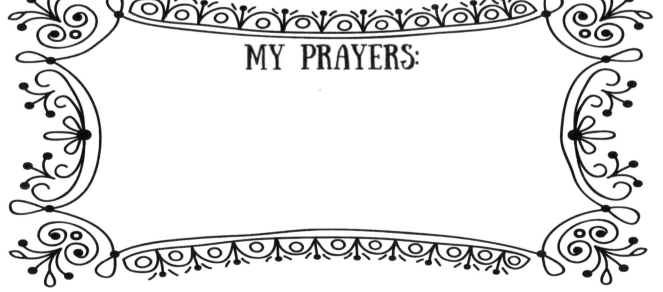

MY PRAYERS:

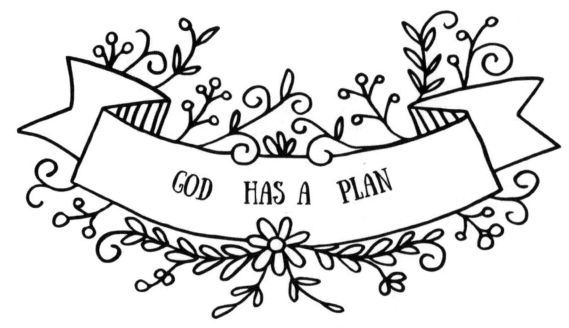

GOD HAS A PLAN

I put my confident trust in the Lord about my pregnancy and the future of my sweet baby. I will seek the Lord, and He will never abandon me and my family.
"AND THOSE WHO KNOW YOUR NAME [WHO HAVE EXPERIENCED YOUR PRECIOUS MERCY] WILL PUT THEIR CONFIDENT TRUST IN YOU, FOR YOU, O LORD, HAVE NOT ABANDONED THOSE WHO SEEK YOU."
PSALM 9:10 AMP

I give God all the glory, who is able to accomplish more than I could ever ask or think.
"NOW ALL GLORY TO GOD, WHO IS ABLE, THROUGH HIS MIGHTY POWER AT WORK WITHIN US, TO ACCOMPLISH INFINITELY MORE THAN WE MIGHT ASK OR THINK."
EPHESIANS 3:20 NLT

I will not worry about things that are out of my control, because God has a perfect plan for me and my family.
"SO DO NOT WORRY ABOUT TOMORROW; FOR TOMORROW WILL WORRY ABOUT ITSELF. EACH DAY HAS ENOUGH TROUBLE OF ITS OWN."
MATTHEW 6:34 AMP

God will not allow me to slip and fall in any area of my life. I give Him all the burdens of my pregnancy, and He takes care of me and my baby.
"GIVE YOUR BURDENS TO THE LORD, AND HE WILL TAKE CARE OF YOU. HE WILL NOT PERMIT THE GODLY TO SLIP AND FALL."
PSALM 55:22 NLT

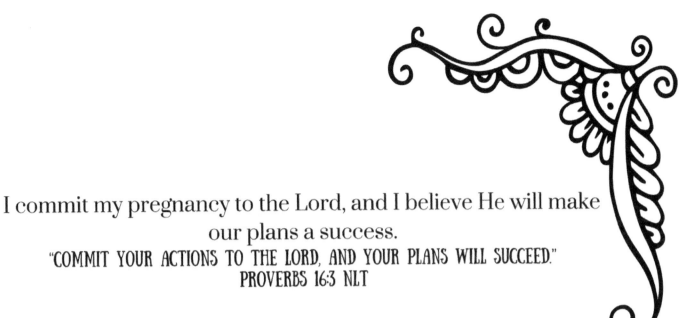

I commit my pregnancy to the Lord, and I believe He will make our plans a success.
"COMMIT YOUR ACTIONS TO THE LORD, AND YOUR PLANS WILL SUCCEED."
PROVERBS 16:3 NLT

God has begun a great work within me, and I am certain He will continue to do great things for me and my family.
"AND I AM CERTAIN THAT GOD, WHO BEGAN THE GOOD WORK WITHIN YOU, WILL CONTINUE HIS WORK UNTIL IT IS FINALLY FINISHED ON THE DAY WHEN CHRIST JESUS RETURNS."
PHILIPPIANS 1:6 NLT

My baby is God's masterpiece that He created. He has good things planned for our future.
"FOR WE ARE GOD'S MASTERPIECE. HE HAS CREATED US ANEW IN CHRIST JESUS, SO WE CAN DO THE GOOD THINGS HE PLANNED FOR US LONG AGO."
EPHESIANS 2:10 NLT

I have complete trust in the Lord, because He guides my steps and puts me in the right place at the right time.
"TRUST IN THE LORD WITH ALL YOUR HEART; DO NOT DEPEND ON YOUR OWN UNDERSTANDING. SEEK HIS WILL IN ALL YOU DO, AND HE WILL SHOW YOU WHICH PATH TO TAKE."
PROVERBS 3:5-6 NLT

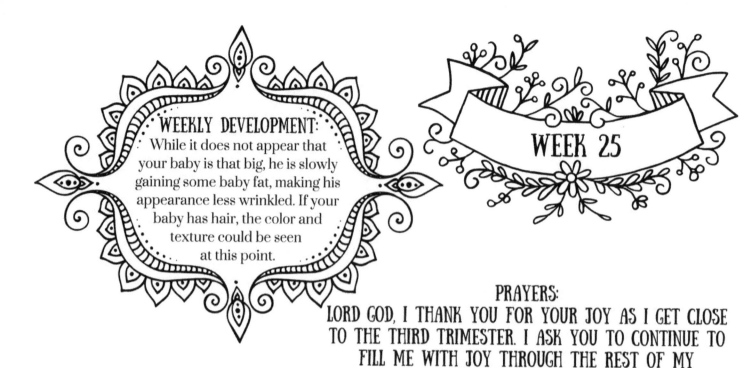

WEEKLY DEVELOPMENT:
While it does not appear that your baby is that big, he is slowly gaining some baby fat, making his appearance less wrinkled. If your baby has hair, the color and texture could be seen at this point.

WEEK 25

PRAYERS:
LORD GOD, I THANK YOU FOR YOUR JOY AS I GET CLOSE TO THE THIRD TRIMESTER. I ASK YOU TO CONTINUE TO FILL ME WITH JOY THROUGH THE REST OF MY PREGNANCY AND DELIVERY.

FATHER GOD, I PRAY OVER MY BABY AS HE GAINS WEIGHT. I PRAY HE WILL FILL OUT WITH ALL OF THE BABY FAT HE NEEDS TO BE HEALTHY AND STRONG WHEN HE ARRIVES.

HEAVENLY FATHER, I PRAY MY DELIVERY WILL COME AT THE EXACT RIGHT TIME. I BELIEVE IT WILL BE A SMOOTH AND EASY DELIVERY, AND THAT ALL THE DOCTORS AND NURSES INVOLVED WILL HAVE WISDOM AS THEY MAKE CHOICES THAT IMPACT ME AND MY NEWBORN.

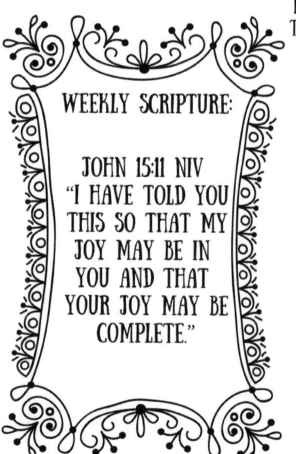

WEEKLY SCRIPTURE:

JOHN 15:11 NIV
"I HAVE TOLD YOU THIS SO THAT MY JOY MAY BE IN YOU AND THAT YOUR JOY MAY BE COMPLETE."

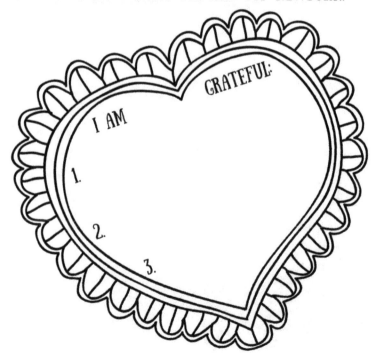

I AM GRATEFUL:

1.

2.

3.

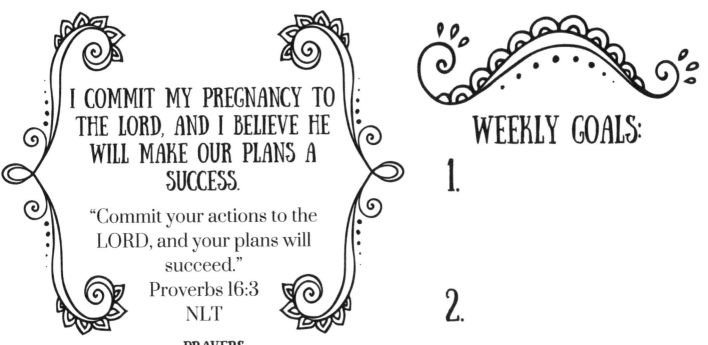

I COMMIT MY PREGNANCY TO THE LORD, AND I BELIEVE HE WILL MAKE OUR PLANS A SUCCESS.

"Commit your actions to the LORD, and your plans will succeed."
Proverbs 16:3
NLT

WEEKLY GOALS:

1.

2.

3.

PRAYERS:

LORD, I THANK YOU FOR MY BABY'S APPEARANCE. AS I EAGERLY AWAIT HIS ARRIVAL, I PRAY THAT EVERY INCH OF IS SKIN WILL FULLY DEVELOP AND THAT HE WILL NOT HAVE TO FACE ANY KIND OF SKIN ISSUES AS HE GROWS UP.

FATHER, TODAY I PRAY AGAINST JAUNDICE. I PRAY ALL THE BABY'S BILIRUBIN LEVELS WILL BE NORMAL AND PREVENT JAUNDICE AT BIRTH.

GRACIOUS GOD, I THANK YOU FOR THE LITTLE THINGS. I THANK YOU THAT MY BABY WILL HAVE BEAUTIFUL HAIR, WHETHER HE HAS HAIR AT BIRTH OR IF IT TAKES MONTHS TO GROW. I THANK YOU FOR THE HAIR THAT WILL PROTECT MY SWEET BABY'S HEAD AND KEEP IT WARM.

MY PRAYERS:

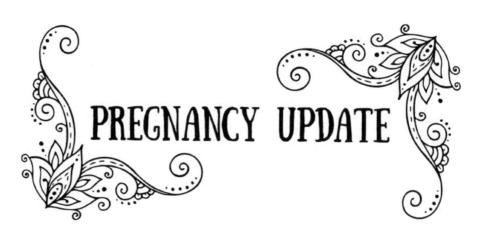

PREGNANCY UPDATE

EMOTIONS I'M FEELING:

_____
_____
_____
_____

PREGNANCY SYMPTOMS:

_____
_____
_____
_____

FOODS:

CAN'T GET ENOUGH:

_____
_____
_____

CAN'T STAND:

_____
_____
_____

FAVORITE PREGNANCY OUTFIT:

_____
_____
_____

NOTES TO MY BABY:

_____
_____
_____
_____

BABY OR BUMP PICTURE

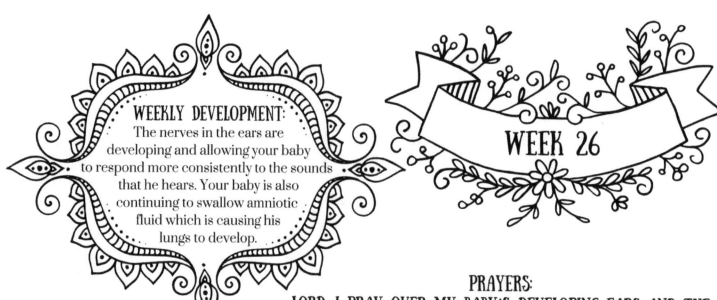

WEEKLY DEVELOPMENT:
The nerves in the ears are developing and allowing your baby to respond more consistently to the sounds that he hears. Your baby is also continuing to swallow amniotic fluid which is causing his lungs to develop.

WEEK 26

PRAYERS:
LORD, I PRAY OVER MY BABY'S DEVELOPING EARS AND THE NERVES WITHIN HIS EARS. I PRAY EVERY SMALL PARTICLE OF THE EARS WILL BE FULLY FUNCTIONING FROM THE DAY MY BABY IS BORN.

LORD GOD, I THANK YOU THAT YOU HAVE GIVEN US THE ABILITY TO HEAR AND THE ABILITY TO HEAR FROM YOU. I WILL LISTEN FOR YOUR VOICE TO KEEP MYSELF AND MY CHILD ON THE RIGHT TRACK.

HEAVENLY FATHER, I PRAY OVER THE LUNGS THAT ARE CONTINUING TO DEVELOP IN MY BABY. I THANK YOU THAT THE LUNGS ARE GETTING THE PRACTICE THEY NEED TO BE ABLE TO SUPPORT MY BABY AFTER BIRTH.

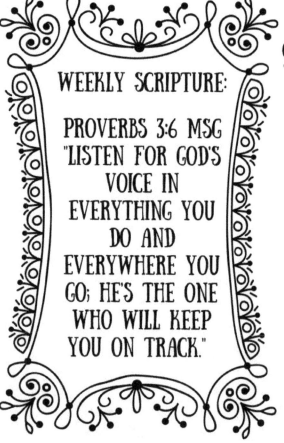

WEEKLY SCRIPTURE:

PROVERBS 3:6 MSG
"LISTEN FOR GOD'S VOICE IN EVERYTHING YOU DO AND EVERYWHERE YOU GO; HE'S THE ONE WHO WILL KEEP YOU ON TRACK."

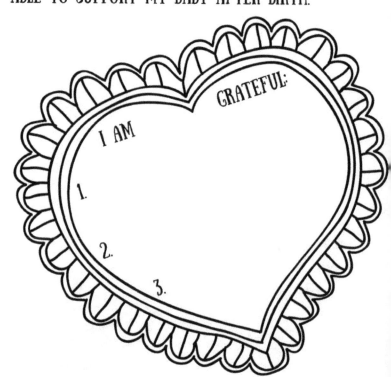

I AM   GRATEFUL:

1.

2.

3.

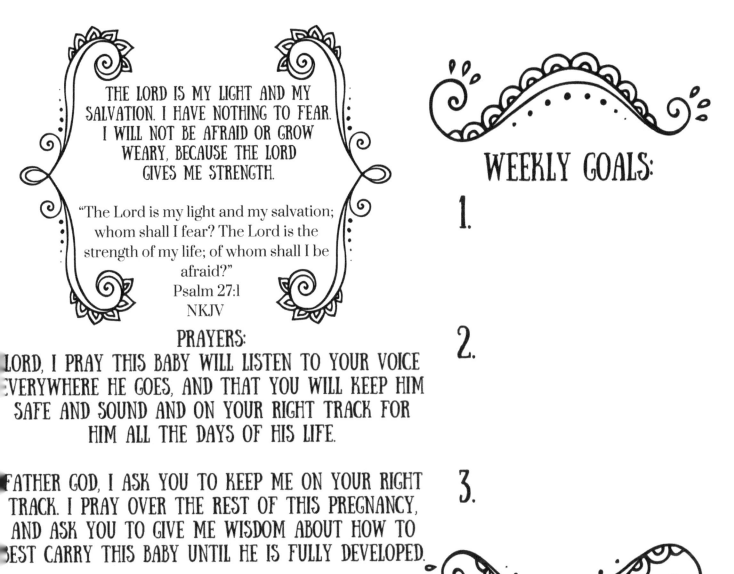

THE LORD IS MY LIGHT AND MY SALVATION. I HAVE NOTHING TO FEAR. I WILL NOT BE AFRAID OR GROW WEARY, BECAUSE THE LORD GIVES ME STRENGTH.

"The Lord is my light and my salvation; whom shall I fear? The Lord is the strength of my life; of whom shall I be afraid?"
Psalm 27:1
NKJV

WEEKLY GOALS:

1.

2.

3.

PRAYERS:

LORD, I PRAY THIS BABY WILL LISTEN TO YOUR VOICE EVERYWHERE HE GOES, AND THAT YOU WILL KEEP HIM SAFE AND SOUND AND ON YOUR RIGHT TRACK FOR HIM ALL THE DAYS OF HIS LIFE.

FATHER GOD, I ASK YOU TO KEEP ME ON YOUR RIGHT TRACK. I PRAY OVER THE REST OF THIS PREGNANCY, AND ASK YOU TO GIVE ME WISDOM ABOUT HOW TO BEST CARRY THIS BABY UNTIL HE IS FULLY DEVELOPED.

LORD, I THANK YOU FOR THE AMNIOTIC FLUID THAT IS HELPING MY BABY'S LUNGS TO DEVELOP. I PRAY MY WOMB WILL CONTINUE TO BE A FERTILE PLACE OF GROWTH AS THE BABY'S DEVELOPMENT CONTINUES.

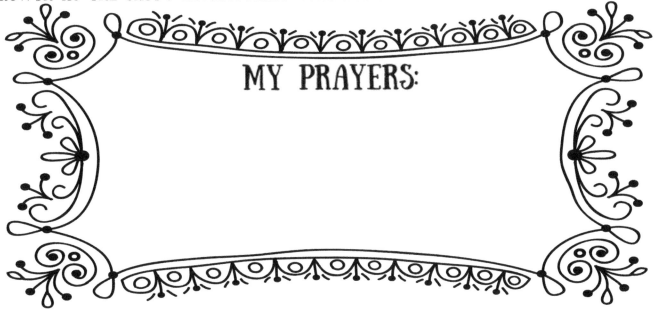

MY PRAYERS:

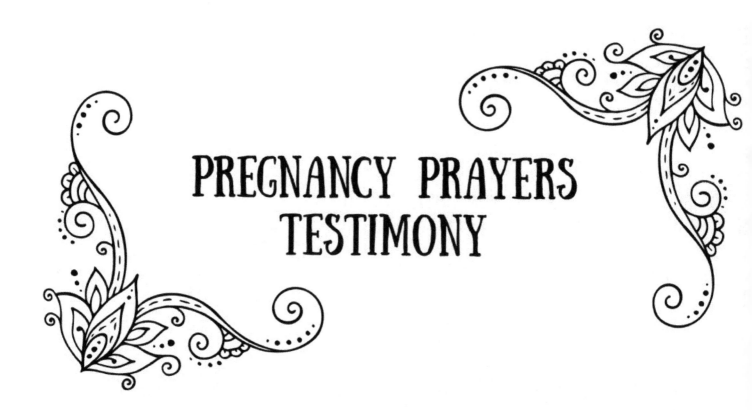

PREGNANCY PRAYERS
TESTIMONY

Pregnancy Prayers is such an awesome daily boost for pregnant women, their friends and family! The daily prayers and encouragements give you daily reminders during the course of your pregnancy that bring great peace and inspiration! And if you aren't pregnant–but you want to be reminded of a friend or family member who is–you can download the app and it reminds you to pray for them!

What a gift! Thank you,
Pregnancy Prayers.
— Youiyiyyyyy (app store testimony)

Download the Pregnancy Prayers app in iTunes and the Google Play stores.

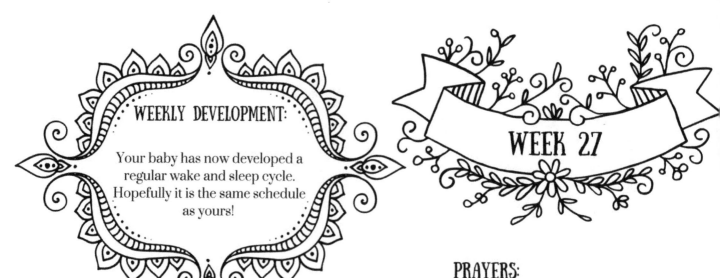

WEEKLY DEVELOPMENT:

Your baby has now developed a regular wake and sleep cycle. Hopefully it is the same schedule as yours!

WEEK 27

PRAYERS:

THANK YOU, LORD, THAT I HAVE MADE IT TO THE THIRD TRIMESTER! I ASK FOR YOUR GRACE TO GET ME THROUGH THIS LAST TRIMESTER! I BELIEVE I HAVE PEACE AND ENERGY THAT PASSES ALL UNDERSTANDING AS I GET READY FOR THE ARRIVAL OF OUR NEW BABY.

DEAR GOD, I THANK YOU THAT THIS BABY HAS DEVELOPED A REGULAR SLEEP CYCLE. I ASK YOU TO HELP THIS BABY TO BE A GOOD SLEEPER AND A SELF-SOOTHER.

HEAVENLY FATHER, I SPEAK OVER THIS BABY AND BELIEVE HE WILL BE A GOOD SLEEPER, AND WILL NOT HAVE NIGHT TERRORS AT ANY POINT WHEN HE SLEEPS.

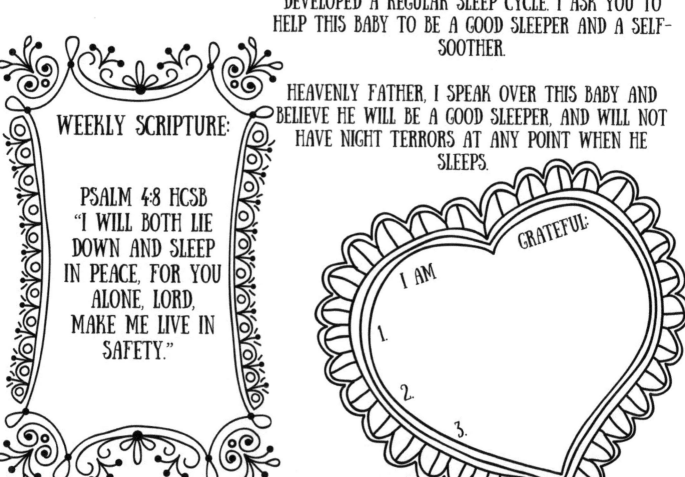

WEEKLY SCRIPTURE:

PSALM 4:8 HCSB
"I WILL BOTH LIE DOWN AND SLEEP IN PEACE, FOR YOU ALONE, LORD, MAKE ME LIVE IN SAFETY."

I AM GRATEFUL:

1.

2.

3.

I AM OVERFLOWING WITH HOPE
FOR MY FAMILY'S FUTURE!
OUR LIVES WILL BE FILLED
WITH GOD'S AMAZING GOODNESS.

"'For I know the plans I have for you,'
says the Lord. 'They are plans for
good and not for disaster, to give you
a future and a hope.'"
Jeremiah 29:11
NLT

WEEKLY GOALS:

1.

PRAYERS:

DEAR LORD, I KNOW HOW IMPORTANT SLEEP IS TO A
MOTHER AND NEW BABY. I ASK THAT THIS BABY NOT
GET HIS DAYS AND NIGHTS CONFUSED AFTER BIRTH,
BUT THAT THE TRANSITION GOING FROM SLEEPING IN
THE WOMB TO SLEEPING IN THIS WORLD WILL BE AN
EASY ONE.

2.

I THANK YOU FOR YOUR SCRIPTURE THAT SAYS I WILL
LIE DOWN AND SLEEP IN PEACE. I ASK FOR YOUR
PEACE TO SLEEP WITHOUT WORRIES ABOUT MY
UPCOMING DELIVERY.

3.

LORD, I ASK YOU TO MAKE THIS CHILD LIVE IN SAFETY
NOW AND THROUGH HIS WHOLE LIFE. WRAP HIM IN
YOUR SAFETY.

MY PRAYERS:

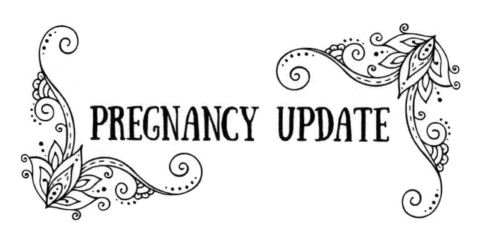

PREGNANCY UPDATE

EMOTIONS I'M FEELING:

_____
_____
_____

PREGNANCY SYMPTOMS:

_____
_____
_____

FOODS:

CAN'T GET ENOUGH: CAN'T STAND:

_____   _____
_____   _____
_____   _____

FAVORITE PREGNANCY OUTFIT:

_____
_____
_____

NOTES TO MY BABY:

_____
_____
_____
_____

BABY OR BUMP PICTURE

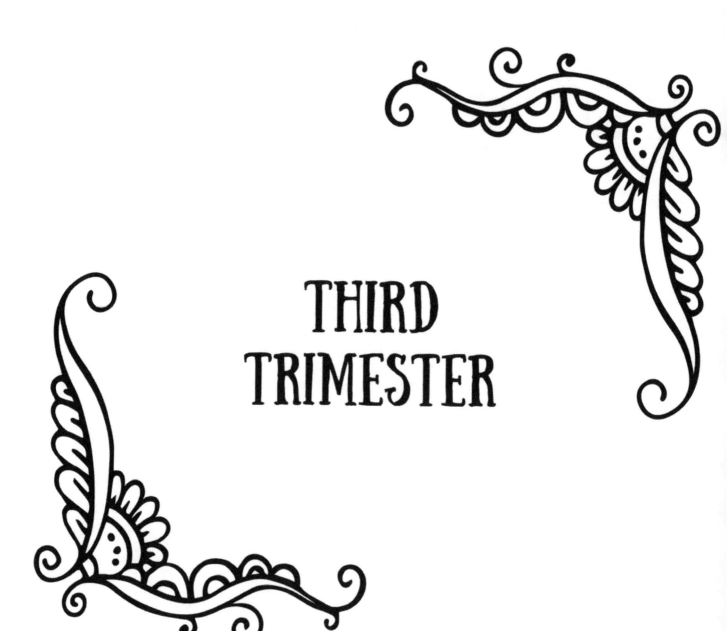

THIRD TRIMESTER

Now stand here and
see the great thing the
LORD
is about to do.
1 Samuel 12:16
NLT

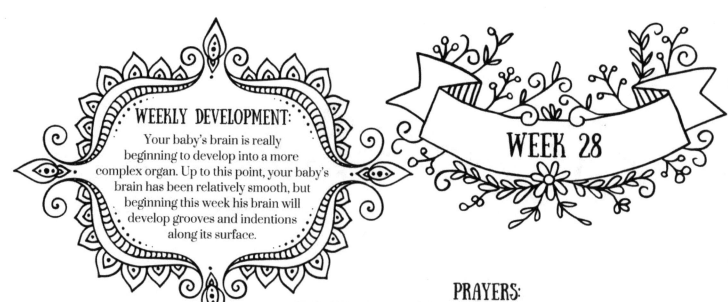

WEEKLY DEVELOPMENT:
Your baby's brain is really beginning to develop into a more complex organ. Up to this point, your baby's brain has been relatively smooth, but beginning this week his brain will develop grooves and indentions along its surface.

WEEK 28

PRAYERS:
FATHER GOD, TODAY I PRAY FOR MY BABY'S BRAIN DEVELOPMENT. I PRAY THAT AS IT BECOMES A MORE COMPLEX ORGAN, IT WILL GROW AND EXPAND TO ITS APPROPRIATE SIZE.

LORD, I PRAY FOR WISDOM FOR THIS BABY. YOUR WORD SAYS THAT IN YOU WE WILL HAVE WISDOM AND STRENGTH, AND I RECEIVE BOTH OF THOSE FOR MY BABY.

THANK YOU, LORD, FOR YOUR WISDOM AND STRENGTH! I PRAY I WILL HAVE WISDOM ABOUT HOW TO RAISE THIS CHILD AND THE STRENGTH TO FOLLOW YOUR PERFECT PLAN.

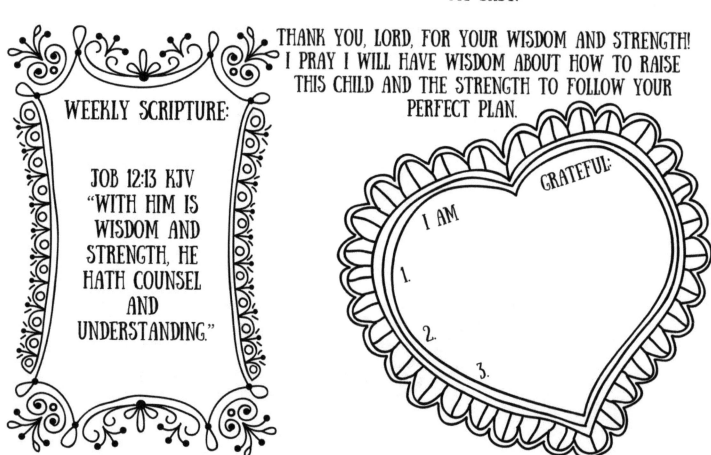

WEEKLY SCRIPTURE:

JOB 12:13 KJV
"WITH HIM IS WISDOM AND STRENGTH, HE HATH COUNSEL AND UNDERSTANDING."

I AM GRATEFUL:
1.
2.
3.

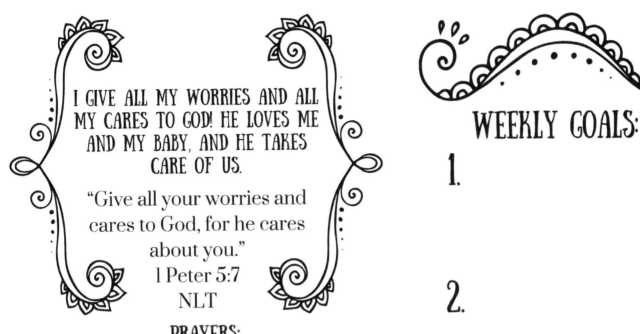

I GIVE ALL MY WORRIES AND ALL MY CARES TO GOD! HE LOVES ME AND MY BABY, AND HE TAKES CARE OF US.

"Give all your worries and cares to God, for he cares about you."
1 Peter 5:7
NLT

WEEKLY GOALS:

1.

2.

3.

PRAYERS:

DEAR LORD, I CONTINUE TO PRAY OVER MY BABY'S BRAIN DEVELOPMENT. I ASK THAT EVERY GROOVE AND INDENTION BE PLACED IN THE RIGHT SPOT TO ENABLE ALL OF THE BRAIN TO FUNCTION COMPLETELY.

HEAVENLY FATHER, I PRAY OVER THE FLUID ON THE BRAIN. I PRAY THAT ONLY THE PRECISE AMOUNT OF FLUID WILL BE LOCATED WITHIN THE SKULL TO SUPPORT THE BRAIN WITH NO EXCESS IN ANY AREA.

LORD, I CONTINUE TO THANK YOU FOR YOUR WISDOM. I ASK THAT EVERY PERSON INVOLVED IN MY DELIVERY WILL HAVE YOUR WISDOM THAT YOU PROMISED IN YOUR WORD.

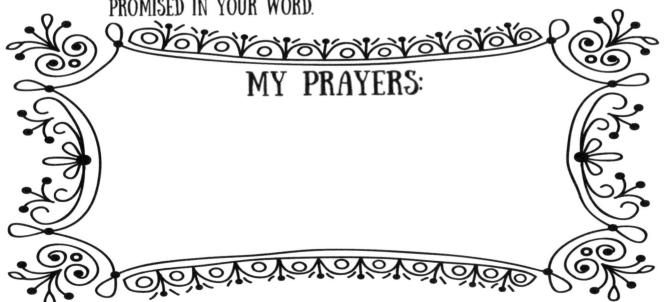

MY PRAYERS:

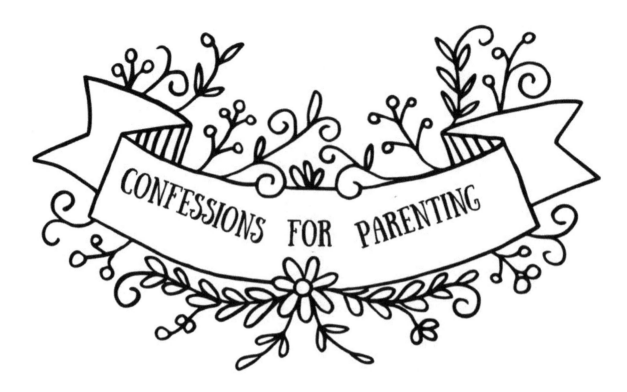

CONFESSIONS FOR PARENTING

My family will always have all we need, because our God will supply all we need and more to be a blessing to others.
"AND GOD WILL GENEROUSLY PROVIDE ALL YOU NEED. THEN YOU WILL ALWAYS HAVE EVERYTHING YOU NEED AND PLENTY LEFT OVER TO SHARE WITH OTHERS."
2 CORINTHIANS 9:8 NLT

My God has not given me a spirit of fear for my family! I have a spirit of power, of love and of a sound mind to be an excellent parent to my children.
"FOR GOD HAS NOT GIVEN US A SPIRIT OF FEAR,
BUT OF POWER AND OF LOVE AND OF A SOUND MIND."
2 TIMOTHY 1:7 NKJV

God, I thank You for the miraculous work you are doing in my baby's body. I trust that You will show me how to be the parent my baby needs to finish the work You have started.
"AND I AM CERTAIN THAT GOD, WHO BEGAN THE GOOD WORK WITHIN YOU,
WILL CONTINUE HIS WORK UNTIL IT IS FINALLY FINISHED ON THE DAY WHEN
CHRIST JESUS RETURNS."
PHILIPPIANS 1:6 NLT

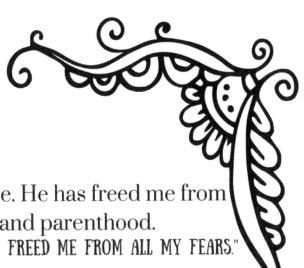

I pray to the Lord, and He answers me. He has freed me from all my fears about pregnancy and parenthood.
"I PRAYED TO THE LORD, AND HE ANSWERED ME. HE FREED ME FROM ALL MY FEARS."
PSALM 34:4 NLT

My heavenly Father will show me exactly how to lead my children down His path. I will be a great parent that sets my children on the path the Lord has planned for them, and they will not leave it in the future.
"DIRECT YOUR CHILDREN ONTO THE RIGHT PATH, AND WHEN THEY ARE OLDER, THEY WILL NOT LEAVE IT."
PROVERBS 22:6 NLT

I am overflowing with hope for my family's future! Our lives will be filled with God's amazing goodness.
"'FOR I KNOW THE PLANS I HAVE FOR YOU,' SAYS THE LORD. 'THEY ARE PLANS FOR GOOD AND NOT FOR DISASTER, TO GIVE YOU A FUTURE AND A HOPE.'"
JEREMIAH 29:11 NLT

I will have faithful love that never ends for my baby. I am full of mercy, just as the Lord's mercies never cease for me.
"THE FAITHFUL LOVE OF THE LORD NEVER ENDS! HIS MERCIES NEVER CEASE."
LAMENTATIONS 3:22 NLT

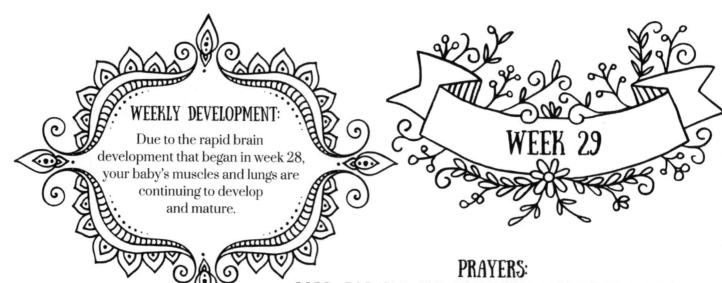

WEEKLY DEVELOPMENT:

Due to the rapid brain development that began in week 28, your baby's muscles and lungs are continuing to develop and mature.

WEEK 29

PRAYERS:

LORD, TODAY I ASK FOR YOUR STRENGTH. I SPEAK STRENGTH OVER MY BODY, AND ASK FOR YOUR HELP AS I CONTINUE THROUGH THIS LAST TRIMESTER.

HEAVENLY FATHER, I THANK YOU FOR ALL THE MUSCLES THAT ARE DEVELOPING IN MY BABY. I AM SO THANKFUL FOR EVERY KICK AND PUNCH I GET TO FEEL AS YOUR MIRACLE IS GROWING INSIDE OF ME.

LORD GOD, I PRAY OVER THE LUNGS THAT ARE CONTINUING TO DEVELOP. I PRAY THAT AS THEY PRACTICE BREATHING, THEY WILL MATURE ENOUGH TO SUPPORT THIS BABY OUT OF THE WOMB.

WEEKLY SCRIPTURE:

I CORINTHIANS 16:13 NIV
"BE ON YOUR GUARD; STAND FIRM IN FAITH; BE COURAGEOUS; BE STRONG."

I AM GRATEFUL:

1.

2.

3.

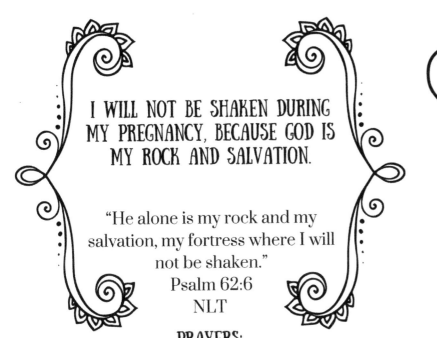

I WILL NOT BE SHAKEN DURING MY PREGNANCY, BECAUSE GOD IS MY ROCK AND SALVATION.

"He alone is my rock and my salvation, my fortress where I will not be shaken."
Psalm 62:6
NLT

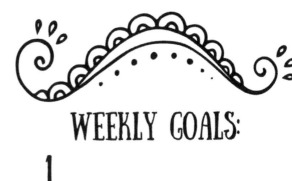

WEEKLY GOALS:

1.

2.

3.

PRAYERS:

FATHER GOD, HELP ME TO STAND FIRM IN FAITH. I PRAY OVER MY BODY AS I CONTINUE TO CARRY THIS CHILD TO FULL TERM, AND STAND IN FAITH THAT DELIVERY WILL NOT BE A TRAUMATIC PROCESS.

TODAY I CONTINUE TO PRAY OVER THE DEVELOPING MUSCLES. I THANK YOU THAT ALL OF THE MUSCLES ARE GROWING AND DEVELOPING JUST AS THEY NEED TO IN ORDER TO BE HIGHLY FUNCTIONING AFTER DELIVERY.

GRACIOUS GOD, I PRAY OVER ALL OF THE MUSCLES IN MY BABY'S LUNGS AS THEY CONTINUE TO GROW AND DEVELOP. I PRAY THE ENTIRE RESPIRATORY SYSTEM WILL BE FULLY FUNCTIONING, AND HAVE THE STRENGTH TO SUPPORT THE BABY AS SOON AS HE IS BORN.

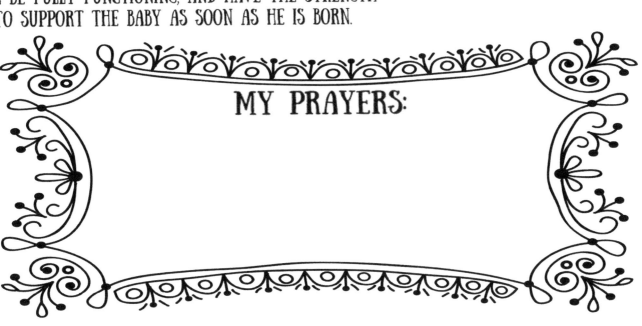

MY PRAYERS:

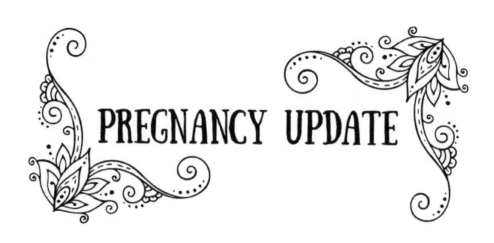

PREGNANCY UPDATE

EMOTIONS I'M FEELING:

_____
_____
_____

PREGNANCY SYMPTOMS:

_____
_____
_____

FOODS:

CAN'T GET ENOUGH: **CAN'T STAND:**

_____   _____
_____   _____
_____   _____

FAVORITE PREGNANCY OUTFIT:

_____
_____
_____

NOTES TO MY BABY:

_____
_____
_____

BABY OR BUMP PICTURE

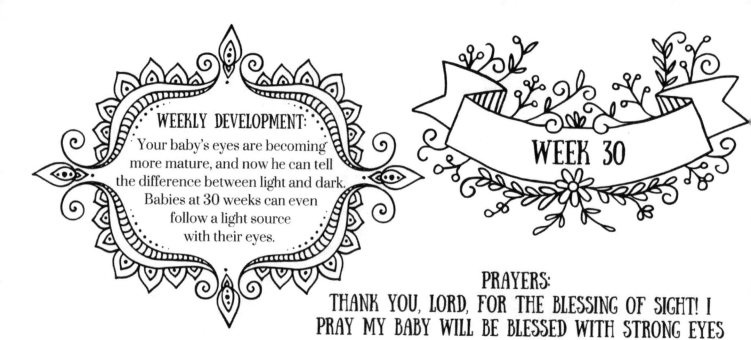

WEEKLY DEVELOPMENT:
Your baby's eyes are becoming more mature, and now he can tell the difference between light and dark. Babies at 30 weeks can even follow a light source with their eyes.

WEEK 30

PRAYERS:
THANK YOU, LORD, FOR THE BLESSING OF SIGHT! I PRAY MY BABY WILL BE BLESSED WITH STRONG EYES FROM THE MOMENT HE IS BORN.

DEAR LORD, I PRAY OVER MY BABY'S EYES AS THEY BEGIN TO TELL THE DIFFERENCE BETWEEN LIGHT AND DARK. I PRAY ALL OF THE MUSCLES IN THE EYE WILL CONTINUE TO DEVELOP AND MATURE.

FATHER GOD, I PRAY OVER MY BABY'S SLEEP PATTERNS. I PRAY HE WILL UNDERSTAND THE DIFFERENCE BETWEEN NIGHT AND DAY, AND NOT HAVE THEM CONFUSED AS HE LEARNS A SLEEP ROUTINE.

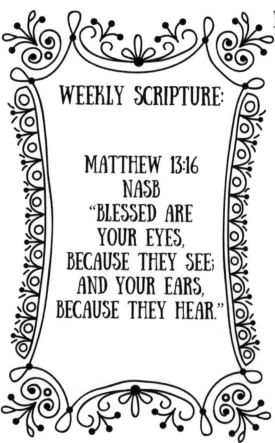

WEEKLY SCRIPTURE:

MATTHEW 13:16 NASB
"BLESSED ARE YOUR EYES, BECAUSE THEY SEE; AND YOUR EARS, BECAUSE THEY HEAR."

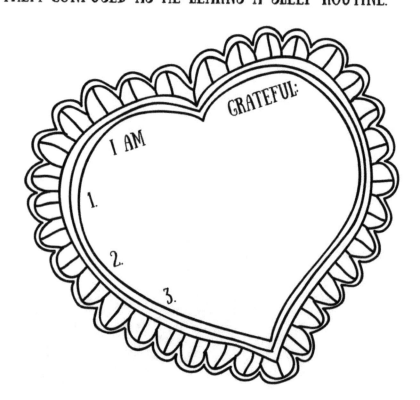

I AM GRATEFUL:

1.

2.

3.

I WILL NOT WORRY ABOUT ANYTHING;
INSTEAD I CHOOSE TO PRAY AND SEEK
GOD'S WISDOM. I AM SO THANKFUL FOR
ALL THAT GOD WILL DO FOR ME AND MY
FAMILY!
"Don't worry about anything;
instead, pray about everything.
Tell God what you need, and thank
him for all he has done."
Philippians 4:6
NLT

WEEKLY GOALS:

1.

2.

3.

PRAYERS:

LORD, I CONTINUE TO PRAY OVER MY BABY'S SLEEP
PATTERNS. I PRAY HE WILL BE A GOOD SLEEPER AND
A SELF-SOOTHER.

LORD GOD, I THANK YOU FOR THE ABILITY TO HEAR
AND ESPECIALLY TO HEAR FROM YOU. I ASK FOR
YOUR WISDOM, AND I WILL HEAR AND LISTEN TO IT
AS I FINISH MY PREGNANCY AND DELIVER THIS BABY.

GRACIOUS GOD, I PRAY OVER MY BABY'S SPIRIT. I
BELIEVE HE HAS A SWEET SPIRIT AND A CALM
NATURE. I PRAY HE WILL BE SWEET AND KIND AND
OBEDIENT ALL THE DAYS OF HIS LIFE.

MY PRAYERS:

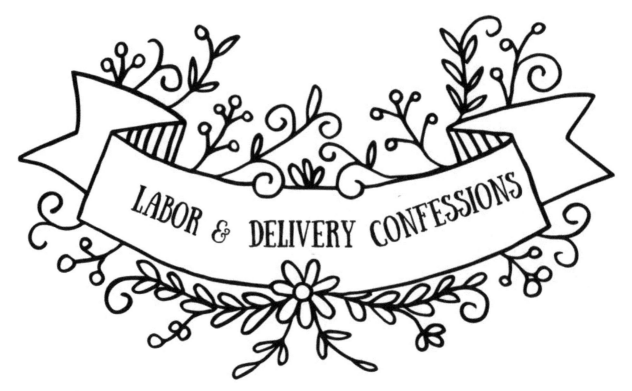

LABOR & DELIVERY CONFESSIONS

I receive God's abundant joy in my pregnancy. I refuse to stress, or have anxiety about my pregnancy and delivery.

"YOU HAVEN'T DONE THIS BEFORE. ASK, USING MY NAME, AND YOU WILL RECEIVE, AND YOU WILL HAVE ABUNDANT JOY."
JOHN 16:24 NLT

My God liberally gives me wisdom as I make choices about my pregnancy and delivery.

"IF ANY OF YOU LACKS WISDOM, LET HIM ASK OF GOD, WHO GIVES TO ALL LIBERALLY AND WITHOUT REPROACH, AND IT WILL BE GIVEN TO HIM."
JAMES 1:5 NKJV

I will not be fearful about labor and delivery, because my God gives me power and self-discipline.

"FOR GOD HAS NOT GIVEN US A SPIRIT OF FEAR AND TIMIDITY, BUT OF POWER, LOVE, AND SELF-DISCIPLINE."
2 TIMOTHY 1:7 NLT

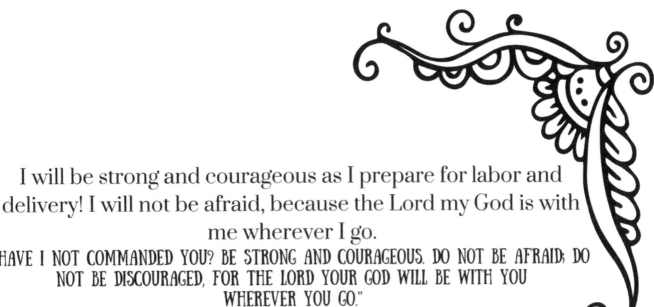

I will be strong and courageous as I prepare for labor and delivery! I will not be afraid, because the Lord my God is with me wherever I go.

"HAVE I NOT COMMANDED YOU? BE STRONG AND COURAGEOUS. DO NOT BE AFRAID; DO NOT BE DISCOURAGED, FOR THE LORD YOUR GOD WILL BE WITH YOU WHEREVER YOU GO."
JOSHUA 1:9 NIV

My Lord who created heaven and earth comes to help me in my pregnancy. He will surely be with me and help me in my labor and delivery.

"MY HELP COMES FROM THE LORD, WHO MADE HEAVEN AND EARTH!"
PSALM 121:2 NLT

God has begun a great work within me throughout my pregnancy. I am certain He will continue His work through my labor and delivery.

"AND I AM CERTAIN THAT GOD, WHO BEGAN THE GOOD WORK WITHIN YOU, WILL CONTINUE HIS WORK UNTIL IT IS FINALLY FINISHED ON THE DAY WHEN CHRIST JESUS RETURNS."
PHILIPPIANS 1:6 NLT

I can do all things through Christ who gives me strength. I will be filled with the Lord's strength and endurance through my labor and delivery!

"I CAN DO ALL THINGS THROUGH CHRIST WHO STRENGTHENS ME."
PHILIPPIANS 4:13 NKJV

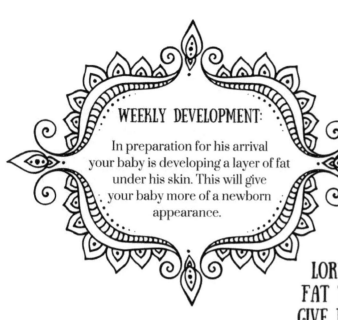

WEEKLY DEVELOPMENT:

In preparation for his arrival your baby is developing a layer of fat under his skin. This will give your baby more of a newborn appearance.

WEEK 31

PRAYERS:

LORD, I THANK YOU FOR THE ESSENTIAL LAYER OF FAT THAT IS DEVELOPING IN MY BABY. I ASK YOU TO GIVE ME WISDOM ABOUT THE CORRECT FOODS TO EAT TO HELP MY BABY GROW HEALTHY AND STRONG.

HEAVENLY FATHER, I THANK YOU FOR YOUR BREATH OF LIFE THAT YOU BREATHED INTO THIS CHILD. I PRAY YOU WILL CONTINUE TO PROTECT MY BABY AS HE GROWS STRONGER EACH DAY.

FATHER GOD, I PRAY FOR YOUR STRENGTH NOW THAT I HAVE LESS THAN 10 WEEKS REMAINING IN MY PREGNANCY. I PRAY FOR THE STRENGTH TO OVERCOME THE ACHES AND PAINS THAT CAN COME WITH THE END OF A PREGNANCY.

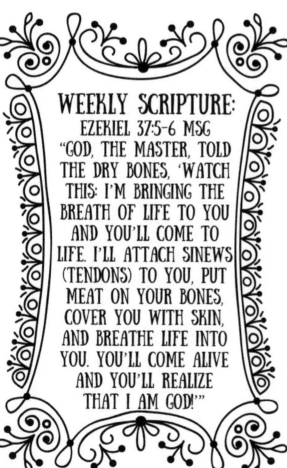

WEEKLY SCRIPTURE:
EZEKIEL 37:5-6 MSG
"GOD, THE MASTER, TOLD THE DRY BONES, 'WATCH THIS: I'M BRINGING THE BREATH OF LIFE TO YOU AND YOU'LL COME TO LIFE. I'LL ATTACH SINEWS (TENDONS) TO YOU, PUT MEAT ON YOUR BONES, COVER YOU WITH SKIN, AND BREATHE LIFE INTO YOU. YOU'LL COME ALIVE AND YOU'LL REALIZE THAT I AM GOD!'"

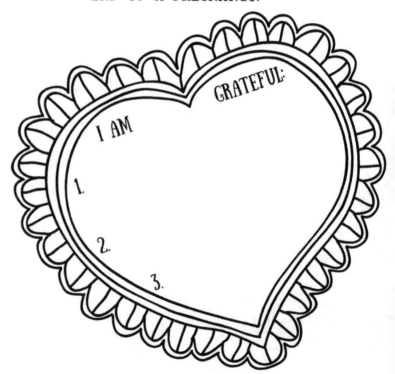

I AM GRATEFUL:
1.
2.
3.

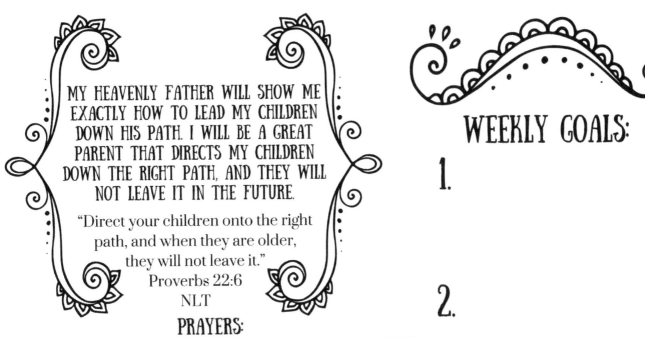

MY HEAVENLY FATHER WILL SHOW ME EXACTLY HOW TO LEAD MY CHILDREN DOWN HIS PATH. I WILL BE A GREAT PARENT THAT DIRECTS MY CHILDREN DOWN THE RIGHT PATH, AND THEY WILL NOT LEAVE IT IN THE FUTURE.

"Direct your children onto the right path, and when they are older, they will not leave it."
Proverbs 22:6
NLT

WEEKLY GOALS:

1.

2.

3.

PRAYERS:

LORD GOD, I THANK YOU THAT YOU ARE GOOD! I PRAY OVER THIS BABY AND THANK YOU FOR MAKING A PERFECT PLAN FOR THE DELIVERY.

LORD, I PRAY OVER ALL OF THE ORGANS THAT ARE DEVELOPING IN MY CHILD, AND I PRAY THAT EVERY SINGLE ORGAN WILL FUNCTION OPTIMALLY FROM THE DAY MY CHILD IS BORN.

GOD, I THANK YOU FOR BREATHING LIFE INTO MY BABY. I PRAY OVER HIS LUNGS AS THEY CONTINUE TO DEVELOP, AND I ASK THAT FROM THE MOMENT HE IS BORN, THEY WILL FUNCTION TO THEIR FULLEST, AND THAT THIS BABY WILL NOT NEED ANY HELP BREATHING.

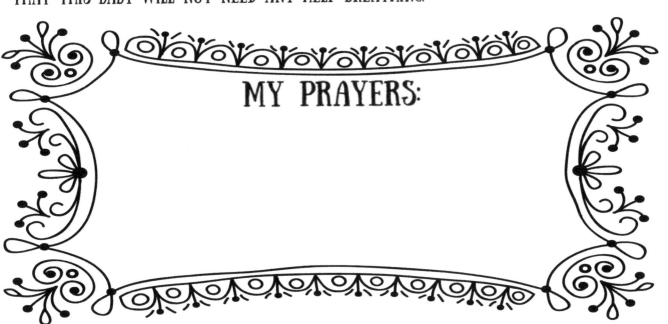

MY PRAYERS:

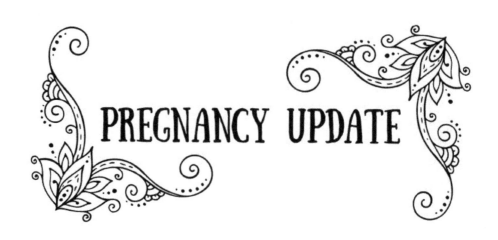

PREGNANCY UPDATE

EMOTIONS I'M FEELING:

_____
_____
_____
_____

PREGNANCY SYMPTOMS:

_____
_____
_____
_____

FOODS:

CAN'T GET ENOUGH:

_____
_____
_____

CAN'T STAND:

_____
_____

FAVORITE PREGNANCY OUTFIT:

_____
_____
_____

NOTES TO MY BABY:

_____
_____
_____
_____

BABY OR BUMP PICTURE

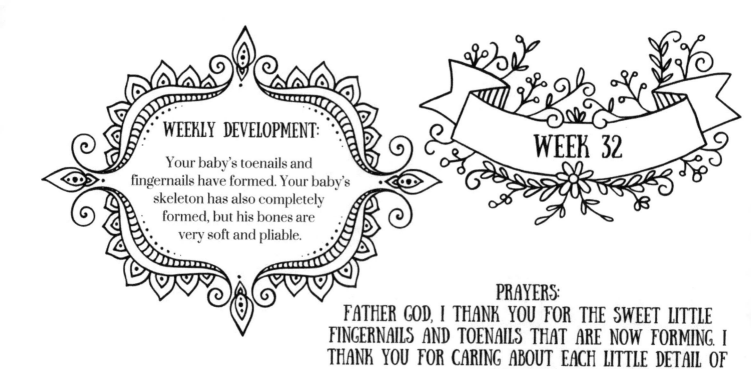

WEEKLY DEVELOPMENT:

Your baby's toenails and fingernails have formed. Your baby's skeleton has also completely formed, but his bones are very soft and pliable.

WEEK 32

PRAYERS:

FATHER GOD, I THANK YOU FOR THE SWEET LITTLE FINGERNAILS AND TOENAILS THAT ARE NOW FORMING. I THANK YOU FOR CARING ABOUT EACH LITTLE DETAIL OF MY CHILD.

HEAVENLY FATHER, I PRAY OVER THE BONES IN THIS CHILD. I PRAY THAT WHILE THEY NEED TO BE SOFT AND PLIABLE FOR DELIVERY, THEY WILL HARDEN AND GROW COMPLETELY WITH MY BABY.

LORD, TODAY I AM GRATEFUL THAT MY BABY WILL HAVE STRONG BONES LIKE YOUR WORD SAYS HE WILL. I PRAY THEY WILL NOT BE BRITTLE OR BREAK EASILY, BUT THEY ARE STRONG LIKE PIECES OF BRASS.

WEEKLY SCRIPTURE:

JOB 40:18 KJ21 "HIS BONES ARE AS STRONG PIECES OF BRASS; HIS BONES ARE LIKE BARS OF IRON."

I AM GRATEFUL:

1.

2.

3.

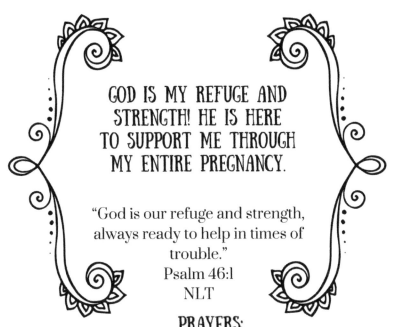

GOD IS MY REFUGE AND
STRENGTH! HE IS HERE
TO SUPPORT ME THROUGH
MY ENTIRE PREGNANCY.

"God is our refuge and strength,
always ready to help in times of
trouble."
Psalm 46:1
NLT

WEEKLY GOALS:

1.

2.

3.

PRAYERS:

LORD GOD, I PRAY OVER THE SKELETON THAT IS
CONTINUING TO FORM. I PRAY THAT EVERY BONE, NO
MATTER HOW SMALL, WILL FORM AND FUSE TOGETHER
CORRECTLY.

FATHER, I PRAY FOR PROTECTION OVER THIS BABY. I
PRAY HE WILL NOT BE ACCIDENT PRONE OR DEAL
WITH INJURIES FREQUENTLY, BUT THAT HE WILL BE
HEALTHY AND STRONG ALL THE DAYS OF HIS LIFE.

LORD, I PRAY OVER THE WORDS THAT COME OUT OF
MY MOUTH ABOUT MY CHILD. HELP ME TO ONLY
SPEAK POSITIVE WORDS OVER MY CHILD AND NOT BE
NEGATIVE. KEEP A GUARD ON MY MOUTH SO THAT I
ONLY SPEAK LIFE AND WHOLENESS OVER MY CHILD
EVERY DAY.

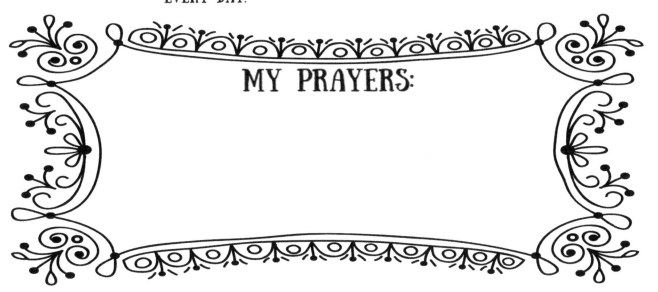

MY PRAYERS:

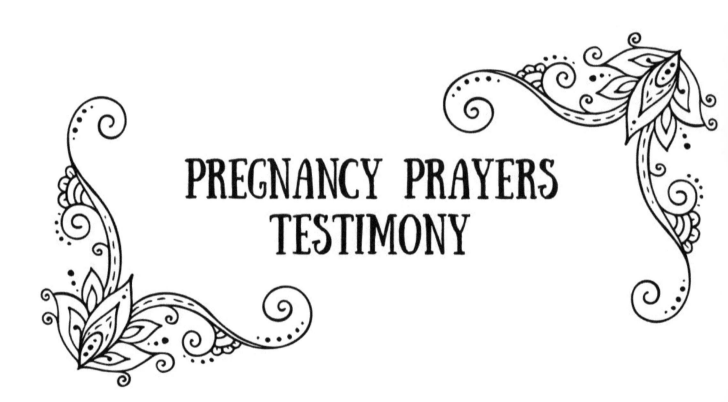

PREGNANCY PRAYERS TESTIMONY

After losing our first baby to hydrocephalous, we were quite cautious about getting excited for our second baby boy.

I downloaded Pregnancy Prayers as soon as it came out and began praying daily for our second baby. We finally reached the point in pregnancy where our baby could survive if he was born, but I was still struggling with worrying about him being born too early like our first baby. Although I knew he could now survive, I wanted him to remain in utero until full term.

That's when I opened my daily prayer from Pregnancy Prayers that said "Lord, I pray my baby will make it to full term. I thank You that if he does come early, he can survive now, but I ask that he stay in the womb until he is completely developed and ready." That prayer brought hope and peace to me as I continued to wait for our perfectly healthy boy to be born. On March 8, 2016, our perfectly healthy baby boy was born at 8 pounds 14 ounces and 22 inches long.

— Chris

Download the Pregnancy Prayers app in iTunes and the Google Play stores.

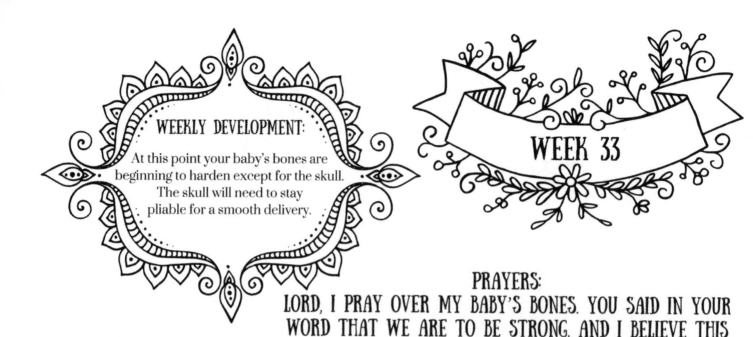

WEEKLY DEVELOPMENT:

At this point your baby's bones are beginning to harden except for the skull. The skull will need to stay pliable for a smooth delivery.

WEEK 33

PRAYERS:

LORD, I PRAY OVER MY BABY'S BONES. YOU SAID IN YOUR WORD THAT WE ARE TO BE STRONG, AND I BELIEVE THIS APPLIES TO MY BABY'S BONES BEING STRONG.

HEAVENLY FATHER, I SPEAK YOUR WORD OVER MY CHILD. YOU SAID YOU WILL BE WITH US WHEREVER WE GO, AND I ASK YOU TO BE WITH MY CHILD WHEREVER HE GOES AS HE GROWS UP.

DEAR GOD, I ASK YOU FOR COURAGE AS I PREPARE TO DELIVER AND HAVE A NEW BABY. I ASK THAT I WILL NOT BE FEARFUL OVER THE DELIVERY PROCESS.

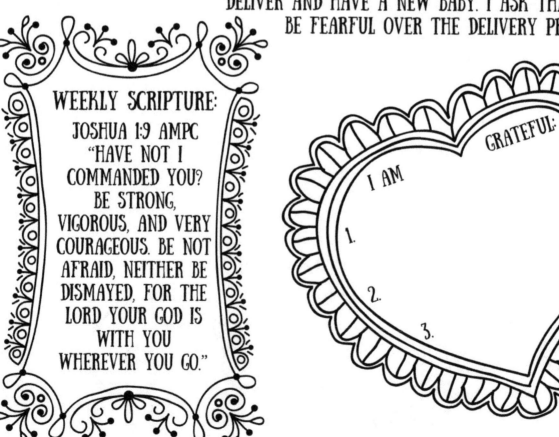

WEEKLY SCRIPTURE:

JOSHUA 1:9 AMPC "HAVE NOT I COMMANDED YOU? BE STRONG, VIGOROUS, AND VERY COURAGEOUS. BE NOT AFRAID, NEITHER BE DISMAYED, FOR THE LORD YOUR GOD IS WITH YOU WHEREVER YOU GO."

I AM GRATEFUL:

1.

2.

3.

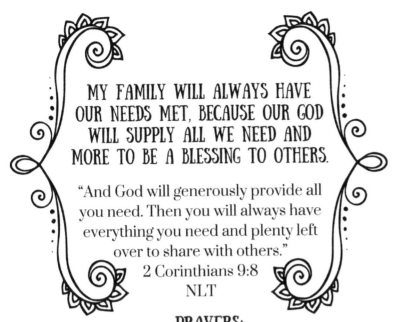

MY FAMILY WILL ALWAYS HAVE OUR NEEDS MET, BECAUSE OUR GOD WILL SUPPLY ALL WE NEED AND MORE TO BE A BLESSING TO OTHERS.

"And God will generously provide all you need. Then you will always have everything you need and plenty left over to share with others."
2 Corinthians 9:8
NLT

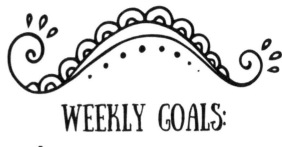

WEEKLY GOALS:

1.

2.

3.

PRAYERS:

TODAY I PRAY OVER MY BABY'S SKULL, AND ASK THAT IT STAY PLIABLE TO ENSURE THAT I HAVE A SMOOTH DELIVERY.

LORD GOD, I CONTINUE TO PRAY OVER THE SKULL TODAY. I ASK THAT AFTER THE DELIVERY, IT WILL CONTINUE TO HARDEN AS IT SHOULD, AND THAT IT WILL NOT BE MISSHAPEN IN ANY WAY.

THANK YOU, LORD, FOR YOUR STRENGTH AND COURAGE AS I CONTINUE IN MY PREGNANCY. I BELIEVE I WILL HAVE ALL THE STRENGTH I NEED TO CONQUER THE DELIVERY PROCESS, AND I WILL NEVER BE DISMAYED AT ANY POINT.

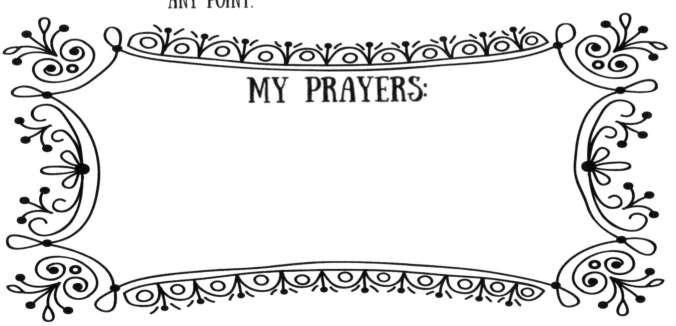

MY PRAYERS:

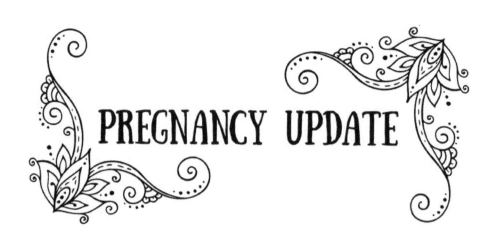

PREGNANCY UPDATE

EMOTIONS I'M FEELING:

_____
_____
_____
_____

PREGNANCY SYMPTOMS:

_____
_____
_____
_____

FOODS:

CAN'T GET ENOUGH:

_____
_____
_____

CAN'T STAND:

_____
_____

FAVORITE PREGNANCY OUTFIT:

_____
_____
_____

NOTES TO MY BABY:

_____
_____
_____
_____

BABY OR BUMP PICTURE

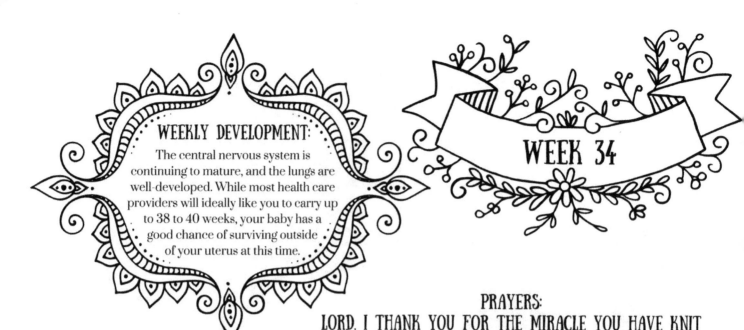

WEEKLY DEVELOPMENT:

The central nervous system is continuing to mature, and the lungs are well-developed. While most health care providers will ideally like you to carry up to 38 to 40 weeks, your baby has a good chance of surviving outside of your uterus at this time.

WEEK 34

PRAYERS:

LORD, I THANK YOU FOR THE MIRACLE YOU HAVE KNIT INSIDE ME. I PRAY MY WOMB WILL CONTINUE TO BE THE PERFECT ENVIRONMENT FOR THIS BABY AS WE PREPARE FOR HIS ARRIVAL IN THE NEXT COUPLE OF WEEKS.

GOD, I PRAY OVER THE CENTRAL NERVOUS SYSTEM AND ALL OF ITS COMPLICATED PARTS. I PRAY OVER EVERY MINUTE DETAIL AS IT CONTINUES TO MATURE AND DEVELOP.

GRACIOUS GOD, I THANK YOU THAT I HAVE MADE IT THIS FAR IN MY PREGNANCY. I AM SO GRATEFUL THAT, JUST LIKE MY BABY, YOU KNIT ME PERFECTLY, AND GAVE MY BODY THE ABILITY TO CARRY A HEALTHY BABY TO FULL TERM.

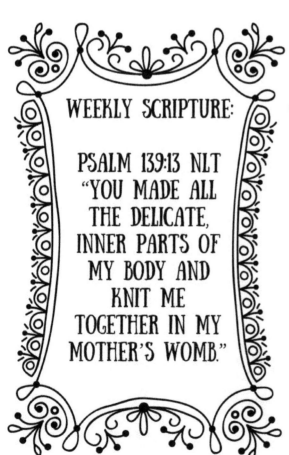

WEEKLY SCRIPTURE:

PSALM 139:13 NLT
"YOU MADE ALL THE DELICATE, INNER PARTS OF MY BODY AND KNIT ME TOGETHER IN MY MOTHER'S WOMB."

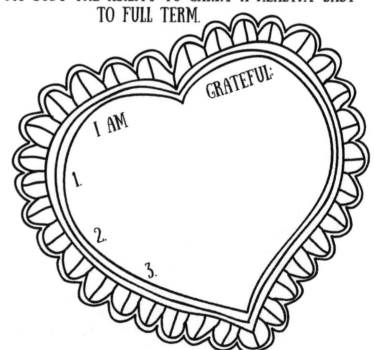

I AM GRATEFUL:

1.

2.

3.

I WILL NOT BE FEARFUL ABOUT LABOR AND DELIVERY, BECAUSE MY GOD GIVES ME POWER TO GET ME THROUGH DELIVERY.

"For God has not given us a spirit of fear and timidity, but of power, love, and self-discipline."
2 Timothy 1:7
NLT

WEEKLY GOALS:

1.

2.

3.

PRAYERS:

FATHER GOD, I PRAY OVER ALL OF THE INNER PARTS OF THIS BABY AS HE FINISHES HIS DEVELOPMENT. I PRAY EVERY PIECE WILL FIT TOGETHER PERFECTLY, AND BE KNIT TOGETHER ACCORDING TO YOUR PERFECT PLAN.

LORD, I PRAY MY BABY WILL MAKE IT TO FULL TERM. I THANK YOU THAT IF HE DOES COME EARLY, HE CAN SURVIVE NOW, BUT I ASK THAT HE STAY IN THE WOMB UNTIL HE IS COMPLETELY DEVELOPED AND READY.

HEAVENLY FATHER, I PRAY OVER ALL SECTIONS OF THE CENTRAL NERVOUS SYSTEM AS THEY CONTINUE TO MATURE. I BELIEVE THAT BOTH THE BRAIN AND THE SPINAL CORD WILL FULLY PROGRESS AND BE COMPLETELY FUNCTIONING.

MY PRAYERS:

HOSPITAL BAG CHECKLIST:

- ♡ Insurance cards
- ♡ Identification cards for mom and dad
- ♡ Phone chargers
- ♡ Camera, video camera and charges
- ♡ Snacks
- ♡ Cash or coins for vending machines
- ♡ Kleenex
- ♡ Baby book and pen
- ♡ Gum and mints
- ♡ Birth plan (if you have one)
- ♡ Entertainment — iPad, laptop, magazines...
- ♡
- ♡
- ♡
- ♡
- ♡

HOSPITAL BAG CHECKLIST FOR MOM:

- ♡ Pajamas you can easily breastfeed in while wearing and a robe
- ♡ Nursing bras and underwear
- ♡ Toothbrush and toothpaste
- ♡ Shower gel, face wash and shower shoes
- ♡ Hairbrush and hair ties
- ♡ Lip balm and lotion
- ♡ Deodorant
- ♡ Glasses and contacts
- ♡ Socks and house shoes
- ♡ Going-home outfit
- ♡
- ♡
- ♡
- ♡
- ♡

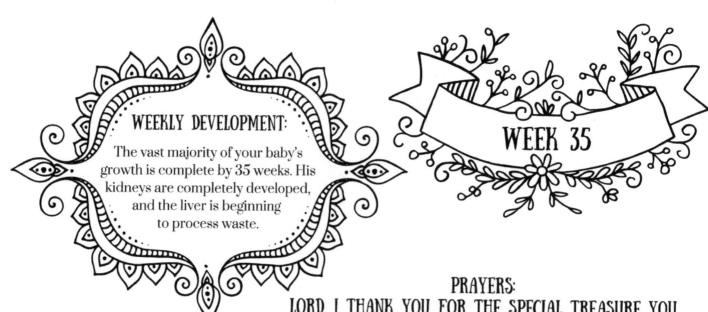

WEEK 35

WEEKLY DEVELOPMENT:
The vast majority of your baby's growth is complete by 35 weeks. His kidneys are completely developed, and the liver is beginning to process waste.

PRAYERS:
LORD, I THANK YOU FOR THE SPECIAL TREASURE YOU HAVE GIVEN ME. I AM SO GRATEFUL THAT MY BABY IS ALMOST FULLY GROWN, AND HE WILL CONTINUE TO GROW STRONG IN THE WOMB.

HEAVENLY FATHER, I PRAY OVER THE KIDNEYS, AND ASK THAT THEY WILL BE FULLY FUNCTIONING ALL THE DAYS OF MY BABY'S LIFE.

DEAR LORD, I THANK YOU FOR THE LIVER. I KNOW IT PLAYS A CRUCIAL ROLE IN PREVENTING JAUNDICE, AND I ASK THAT IT WILL BE ABLE TO PROCESS ALL OF THE WASTE IT NEEDS TO PREVENT JAUNDICE.

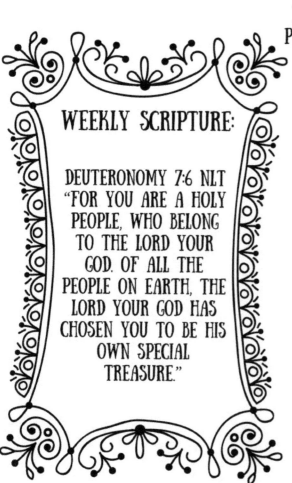

WEEKLY SCRIPTURE:

DEUTERONOMY 7:6 NLT
"FOR YOU ARE A HOLY PEOPLE, WHO BELONG TO THE LORD YOUR GOD. OF ALL THE PEOPLE ON EARTH, THE LORD YOUR GOD HAS CHOSEN YOU TO BE HIS OWN SPECIAL TREASURE."

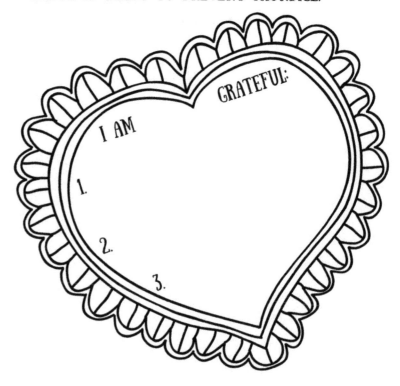

I AM GRATEFUL:

1.

2.

3.

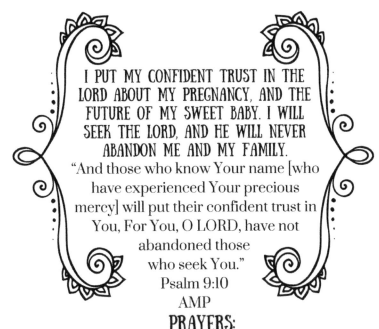

I PUT MY CONFIDENT TRUST IN THE LORD ABOUT MY PREGNANCY, AND THE FUTURE OF MY SWEET BABY. I WILL SEEK THE LORD, AND HE WILL NEVER ABANDON ME AND MY FAMILY.

"And those who know Your name [who have experienced Your precious mercy] will put their confident trust in You, For You, O LORD, have not abandoned those who seek You."

Psalm 9:10
AMP

PRAYERS:

FATHER, I PRAY OVER MY BODY. I ASK FOR YOUR HELP AND WISDOM AS I CARRY THIS BABY TO FULL TERM. GIVE ME WISDOM ABOUT HOW TO CARE FOR MYSELF AND MY GROWING CHILD.

DEAR GOD, I PRAY FOR YOUR COMFORT AS I PREPARE TO DELIVER. I ASK THAT IT WILL NOT BE TRAUMATIC, BUT THAT IT WILL BE A STRESS-FREE DELIVERY.

GRACIOUS GOD, I THANK YOU THAT YOU CREATED A SYSTEM TO ALLOW OUR BODIES TO PROCESS WASTE, AND KEEP US FROM HARM. I PRAY OVER THE LIVER AND THE KIDNEYS AS THEY BEGIN TO FUNCTION, AND ASK THAT THEY WILL FULLY DEVELOP AND WORK PROPERLY AT ALL TIMES.

WEEKLY GOALS:

1.

2.

3.

MY PRAYERS:

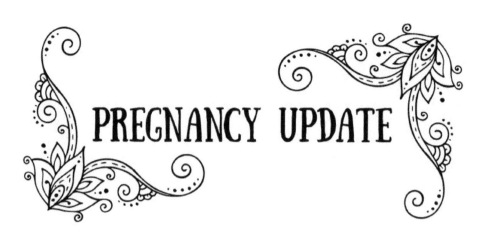

PREGNANCY UPDATE

EMOTIONS I'M FEELING:

_____
_____
_____
_____

PREGNANCY SYMPTOMS:

_____
_____
_____
_____

FOODS:

CAN'T GET ENOUGH: **CAN'T STAND:**

_____   _____
_____   _____
_____   _____

FAVORITE PREGNANCY OUTFIT:

_____
_____
_____

NOTES TO MY BABY:

_____
_____
_____
_____

BABY OR BUMP
PICTURE

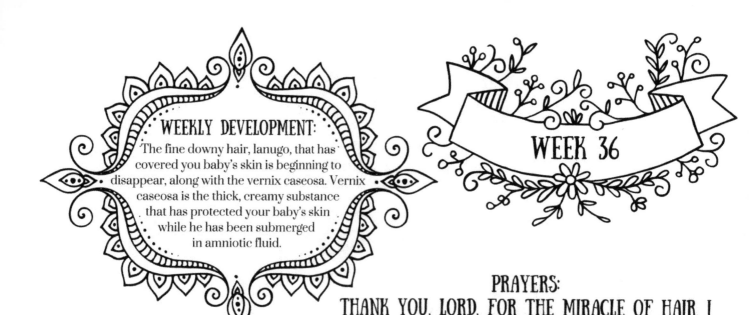

WEEKLY DEVELOPMENT:

The fine downy hair, lanugo, that has covered you baby's skin is beginning to disappear, along with the vernix caseosa. Vernix caseosa is the thick, creamy substance that has protected your baby's skin while he has been submerged in amniotic fluid.

WEEK 36

PRAYERS:

THANK YOU, LORD, FOR THE MIRACLE OF HAIR. I THANK YOU THAT IT HAS BEEN PROTECTING MY BABY FOR WEEKS. I ASK FOR YOUR CONTINUED PROTECTION OVER MY BABY AS HE CONTINUES TO DEVELOP.

LORD, TODAY I PRAY OVER MY BABY'S SKIN. I PRAY OVER THE CREAMY SUBSTANCE THAT IS DISAPPEARING, AND OVER THE NEW SKIN THAT IS CONTINUING TO DEVELOP.

TODAY I PRAY AGAINST ALL SKIN ISSUES. I BELIEVE THIS BABY WILL NOT DEAL WITH CRADLE CAP OR HAVE ANY OTHER SKIN ISSUES AS HE CONTINUES TO GROW IN THE WOMB.

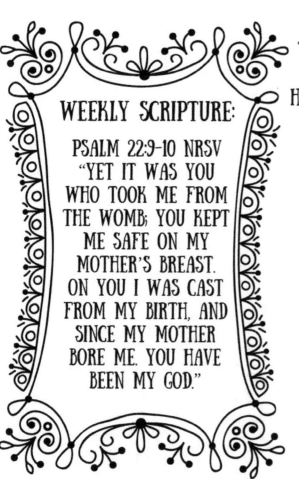

WEEKLY SCRIPTURE:

PSALM 22:9-10 NRSV
"YET IT WAS YOU WHO TOOK ME FROM THE WOMB; YOU KEPT ME SAFE ON MY MOTHER'S BREAST. ON YOU I WAS CAST FROM MY BIRTH, AND SINCE MY MOTHER BORE ME. YOU HAVE BEEN MY GOD."

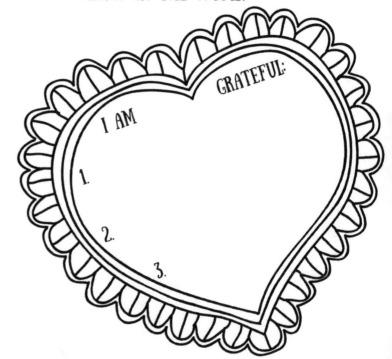

I AM GRATEFUL:

1.

2.

3.

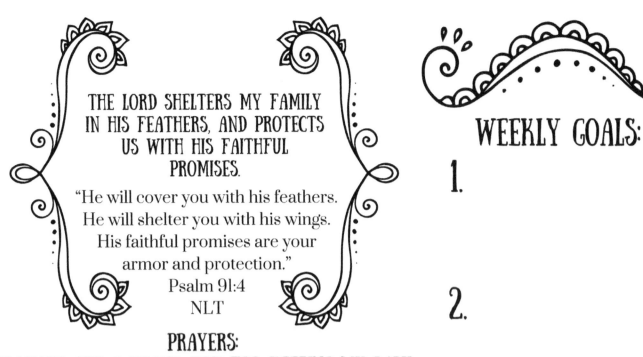

THE LORD SHELTERS MY FAMILY IN HIS FEATHERS, AND PROTECTS US WITH HIS FAITHFUL PROMISES.

"He will cover you with his feathers. He will shelter you with his wings. His faithful promises are your armor and protection."

Psalm 91:4
NLT

WEEKLY GOALS:

1.

2.

3.

PRAYERS:

GRACIOUS GOD, I THANK YOU FOR KEEPING MY BABY SAFE ONCE HE IS OUT OF THE WOMB. KEEP HIM SAFE IN MY ARMS FROM THE MOMENT HE IS BORN.

LORD GOD, I PRAY OVER LABOR AND DELIVERY. I THANK YOU FOR YOUR PERFECT TIMING, AND PRAY THAT MY DELIVERY WILL BE FULL OF PEACE AND NOT ANXIETY.

FATHER GOD, I CONTINUE TO PRAY OVER MY BABY'S SKIN. I PRAY THAT AS IT CONTINUES TO DEVELOP AFTER BIRTH, IT WILL ADJUST TO THE NEW ENVIRONMENT EASILY AND WITHOUT PROBLEMS.

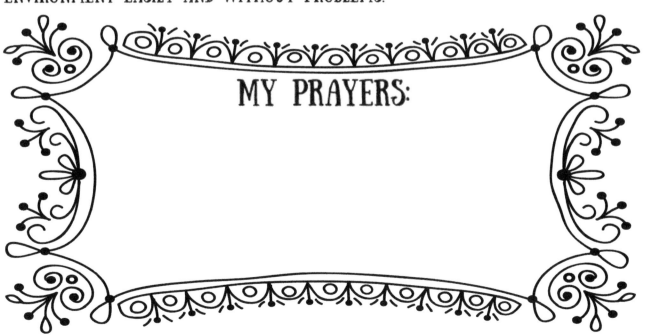

MY PRAYERS:

HOSPITAL BAG CHECKLIST
FOR DAD:

♡ Change of clothes

♡ Socks and underwear

♡ Toothbrush and toothpaste

♡ Shower gel, face wash and shower shoes

♡ Pillow and blanket

♡ Lip balm and lotion

♡ Deodorant

♡ Glasses and contacts

♡ Socks and house shoes

♡ Going-home outfit

♡

♡

♡

♡

♡

146

HOSPITAL BAG CHECKLIST
FOR BABY:

♡ 2 pairs of sleeper pajamas — newborn

♡ 2 pairs of sleeper pajamas — premie

♡ Premie or newborn going-home outfit

♡ Outfit and blanket for pictures

♡ Baby hat or bow

♡ Mittens and socks

♡ Swaddle blankets

♡ Carseat

♡ Burp cloths

♡ Breastfeeding pillow

♡ Outfits for your hospital stay — newborn and premie size

♡

♡

♡

♡

♡

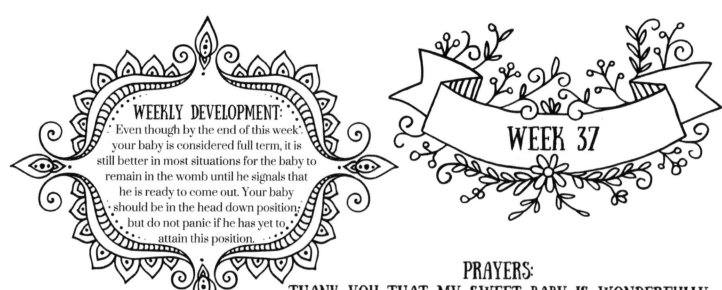

WEEKLY DEVELOPMENT:
Even though by the end of this week your baby is considered full term, it is still better in most situations for the baby to remain in the womb until he signals that he is ready to come out. Your baby should be in the head down position, but do not panic if he has yet to attain this position.

WEEK 37

PRAYERS:
THANK YOU THAT MY SWEET BABY IS WONDERFULLY MADE! I AM INCREDIBLY GRATEFUL FOR THIS PREGNANCY, AND ASK YOU TO CONTINUE TO GIVE ME STRENGTH THROUGH THESE LAST WEEKS.

LORD, I PRAY THAT MY BABY IS IN THE RIGHT POSITION TO DELIVER. I ASK THAT IF HE'S NOT THERE YET, YOU WILL HELP TO GET HIM IN THE CORRECT POSITION BEFORE DELIVERY.

DEAR LORD, I THANK YOU THAT WE HAVE MADE IT TO FULL TERM! I KNOW YOU HAVE THE PERFECT BIRTHDAY FOR MY BABY, AND I AM EXCITED FOR THAT DAY TO COME.

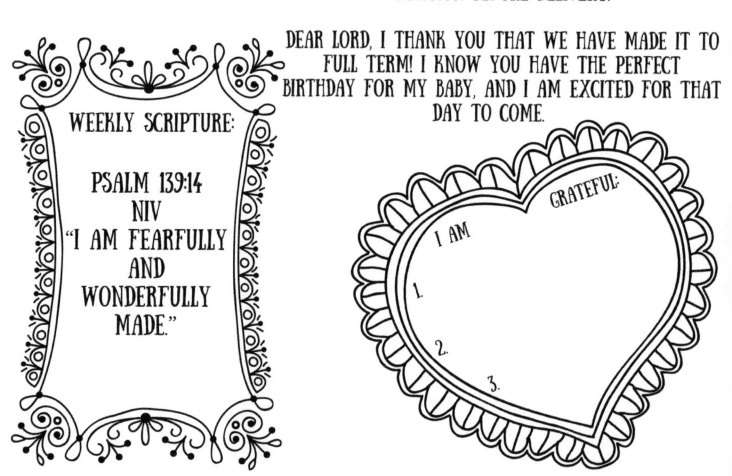

WEEKLY SCRIPTURE:

PSALM 139:14
NIV
"I AM FEARFULLY AND WONDERFULLY MADE."

I AM GRATEFUL:

1.

2.

3.

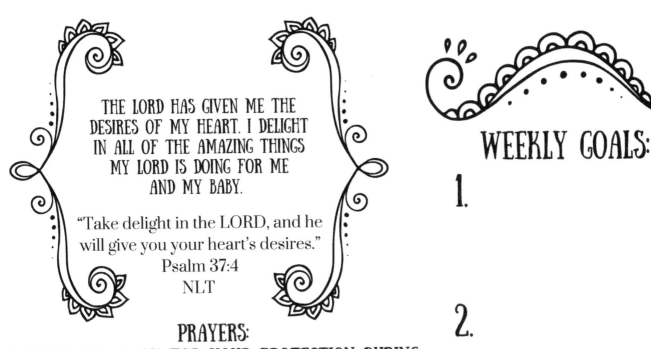

THE LORD HAS GIVEN ME THE DESIRES OF MY HEART. I DELIGHT IN ALL OF THE AMAZING THINGS MY LORD IS DOING FOR ME AND MY BABY.

"Take delight in the LORD, and he will give you your heart's desires."
Psalm 37:4
NLT

WEEKLY GOALS:

1.

2.

3.

PRAYERS:

FATHER GOD, I ASK FOR YOUR PROTECTION DURING ᴅLIVERY FOR ME AND MY BABY. I ASK YOU TO WATCH ᴠER AND PROTECT BOTH OF US THROUGH THE ENTIRE PROCESS.

ᵀODAY I THANK YOU FOR THE DOCTORS, NURSES AND ᴍIDWIVES WHO WILL BE INVOLVED IN DELIVERY. I ASK FOR WISDOM FOR EVERYONE WHO IS HELPING WITH DELIVERY.

ᴇAR FATHER, I THANK YOU THAT YOU HAVE GIVEN ME ᵀHE STRENGTH TO CARRY THIS BABY TO FULL TERM. I ᴀSK FOR YOUR CONTINUED HELP IN THESE LAST FEW WEEKS AS WE PREPARE FOR OUR NEW BABY.

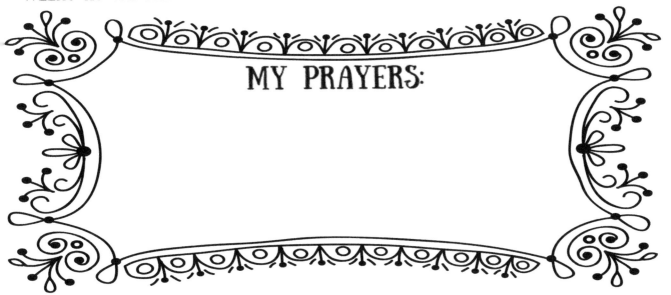

MY PRAYERS:

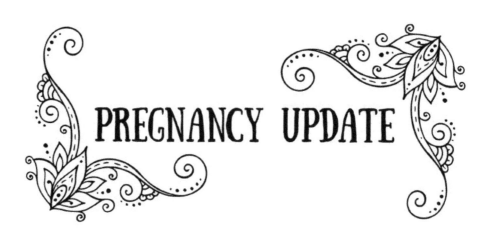

PREGNANCY UPDATE

EMOTIONS I'M FEELING:

_____
_____
_____
_____

PREGNANCY SYMPTOMS:

_____
_____
_____
_____

FOODS:

CAN'T GET ENOUGH:

_____
_____
_____

CAN'T STAND:

_____
_____
_____

FAVORITE PREGNANCY OUTFIT:

_____
_____
_____

NOTES TO MY BABY:

_____
_____
_____
_____

BABY OR BUMP PICTURE

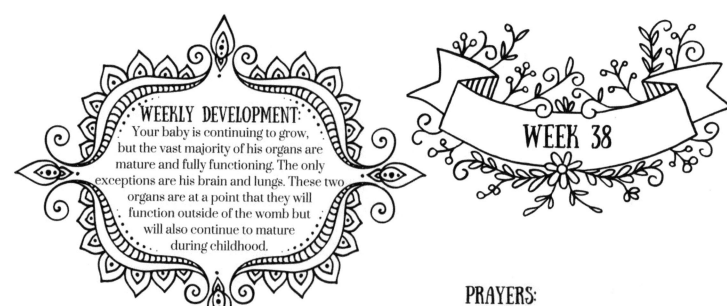

WEEKLY DEVELOPMENT:
Your baby is continuing to grow, but the vast majority of his organs are mature and fully functioning. The only exceptions are his brain and lungs. These two organs are at a point that they will function outside of the womb but will also continue to mature during childhood.

WEEK 38

PRAYERS:
LORD, I THANK YOU THAT MY BABY HAS HAD 38 WEEKS TO GROW AND DEVELOP IN THE WOMB. I PRAY YOU WILL CONTINUE TO BLESS MY LAST WEEKS OF PREGNANCY.

FATHER GOD, I CONTINUE TO PRAY OVER ALL OF MY BABY'S ORGANS, AND THAT EACH ONE WILL BE FULLY FUNCTIONING FROM THE DAY HE IS BORN.

TODAY I PRAY THAT MY CHILD WILL TEACH OTHERS BY HIS LIFE, AND THAT HE WILL ALWAYS WALK IN LOVE AND INTEGRITY.

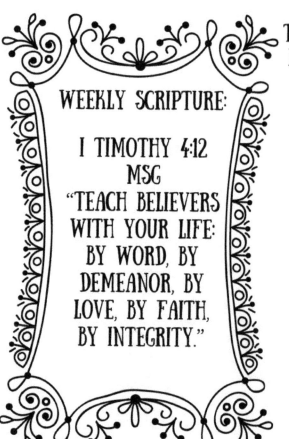

WEEKLY SCRIPTURE:

I TIMOTHY 4:12 MSG
"TEACH BELIEVERS WITH YOUR LIFE: BY WORD, BY DEMEANOR, BY LOVE, BY FAITH, BY INTEGRITY."

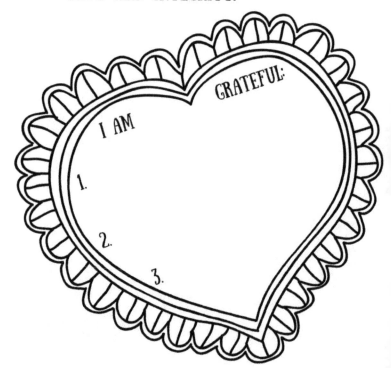

I AM GRATEFUL:

1.

2.

3.

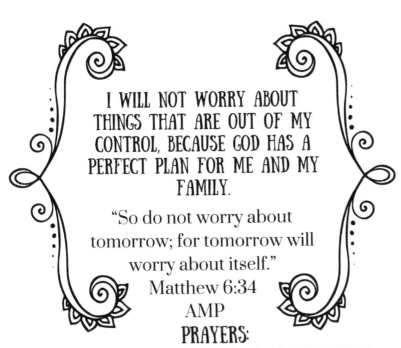

I WILL NOT WORRY ABOUT THINGS THAT ARE OUT OF MY CONTROL, BECAUSE GOD HAS A PERFECT PLAN FOR ME AND MY FAMILY.

"So do not worry about tomorrow; for tomorrow will worry about itself."
Matthew 6:34
AMP

PRAYERS:
DEAR LORD, I PRAY OVER THE CONTINUED DEVELOPMENT OF THE LUNGS. I PRAY THEY WILL BE STRONG WHEN MY BABY IS BORN, AND CONTINUE TO GROW STRONGER EVERY DAY.

THANK YOU, LORD, FOR MY BABY'S BRAIN. I KNOW IT WILL CONTINUE TO GROW AND DEVELOP WITH MY CHILD, AND I THANK YOU THAT IT WILL FULLY DEVELOP AND FUNCTION OPTIMALLY.

HEAVENLY FATHER, I PRAY OVER THE LIVER AND ITS FUNCTION IN KEEPING MY BABY FROM HAVING JAUNDICE. I PRAY IT WILL FUNCTION COMPLETELY AT DELIVERY TO AVOID JAUNDICE AND OTHER COMPLICATIONS.

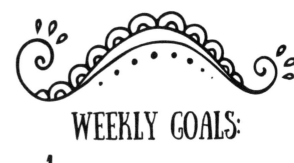

WEEKLY GOALS:

1.

2.

3.

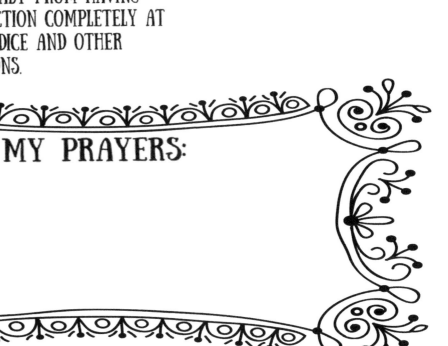

MY PRAYERS:

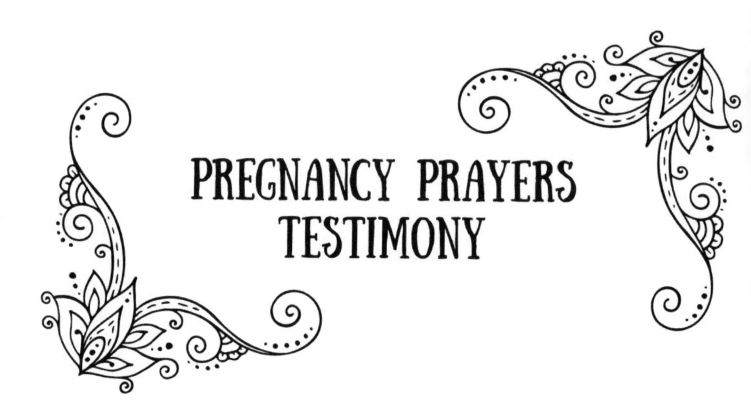

PREGNANCY PRAYERS
TESTIMONY

I, too, had been searching for scriptures to pray over my baby. The Lord has been faithful in providing my husband and I with what to say, but the Pregnancy Prayers app came just in time! With just two weeks to go it's awesome to have the right words to speak for an on-time and perfect delivery.

God is so good! Thank you, Ashley, for this beautiful app!

— Reneelepage (app store testimony)

Download the Pregnancy Prayers app in iTunes and the Google Play stores.

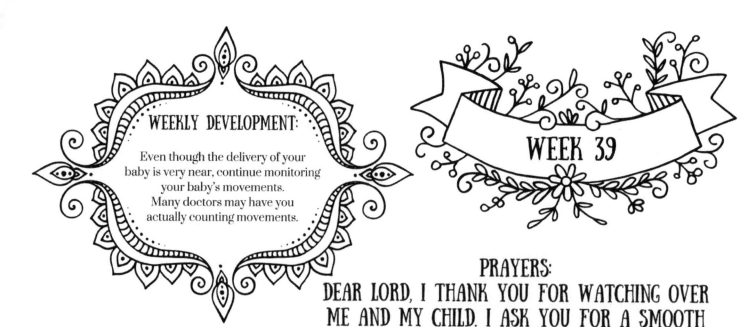

WEEKLY DEVELOPMENT:

Even though the delivery of your baby is very near, continue monitoring your baby's movements. Many doctors may have you actually counting movements.

WEEK 39

PRAYERS:
DEAR LORD, I THANK YOU FOR WATCHING OVER ME AND MY CHILD. I ASK YOU FOR A SMOOTH AND EASY DELIVERY.

FATHER GOD, I CONTINUE TO PRAY OVER ALL OF MY BABY'S ORGANS, AND I PRAY THAT EVERY ORGAN WILL FUNCTION OPTIMALLY FROM THE DAY HE'S BORN.

LORD, TODAY I ASK YOU FOR PEACE AS I PREPARE TO DELIVER AND CARE FOR THIS NEW BABY. I ASK FOR YOUR STRENGTH THROUGH THE DELIVERY, AND THAT THE BABY WILL COME OUT HEALTHY AND STRONG.

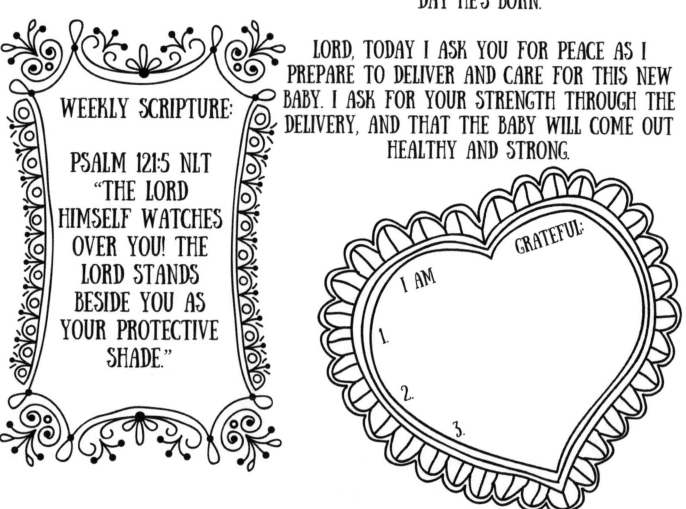

WEEKLY SCRIPTURE:

PSALM 121:5 NLT
"THE LORD HIMSELF WATCHES OVER YOU! THE LORD STANDS BESIDE YOU AS YOUR PROTECTIVE SHADE."

I AM GRATEFUL:
1.
2.
3.

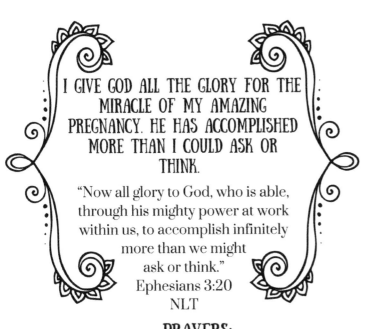

I GIVE GOD ALL THE GLORY FOR THE MIRACLE OF MY AMAZING PREGNANCY. HE HAS ACCOMPLISHED MORE THAN I COULD ASK OR THINK.

"Now all glory to God, who is able, through his mighty power at work within us, to accomplish infinitely more than we might ask or think."
Ephesians 3:20 NLT

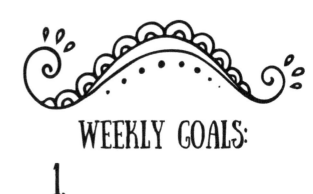

WEEKLY GOALS:

1.

2.

3.

PRAYERS:

THANK YOU, LORD, FOR ALL OF THE MOVEMENT I HAVE BEEN BLESSED TO FEEL FROM THIS BABY. I PRAY THE MOVEMENTS CONTINUE AS THIS BABY GETS STRONGER AND READY TO MAKE HIS APPEARANCE.

GRACIOUS GOD, I AM SO THANKFUL I HAVE MADE IT TO FULL TERM WITH MY BABY. I KNOW YOU HAVE A PERFECT DELIVERY DATE, AND I REST IN YOUR PEACE AS THAT DAY APPROACHES.

TODAY I PRAY THAT MY BABY IS READY FOR DELIVERY AND THAT HE IS IN THE RIGHT POSITION, AND COMPLETELY READY TO COME OUT OF THE WOMB.

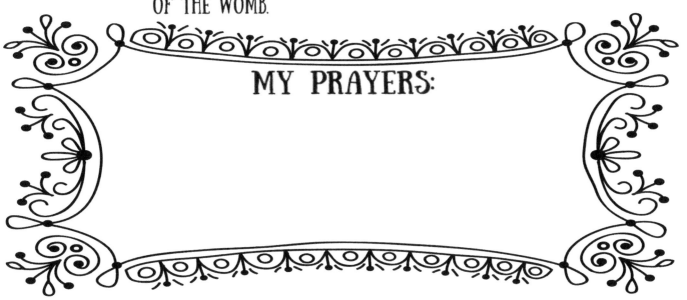

MY PRAYERS:

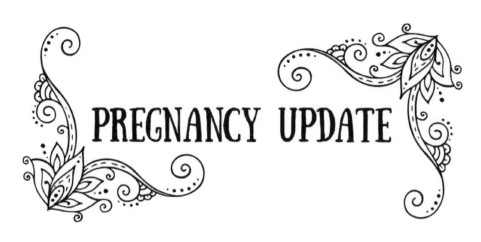

PREGNANCY UPDATE

EMOTIONS I'M FEELING:

_____
_____
_____
_____

PREGNANCY SYMPTOMS:

_____
_____
_____
_____

FOODS:

CAN'T GET ENOUGH:

_____
_____
_____

CAN'T STAND:

_____
_____
_____

FAVORITE PREGNANCY OUTFIT:

_____
_____
_____
_____

NOTES TO MY BABY:

_____
_____
_____
_____

BABY OR BUMP
PICTURE

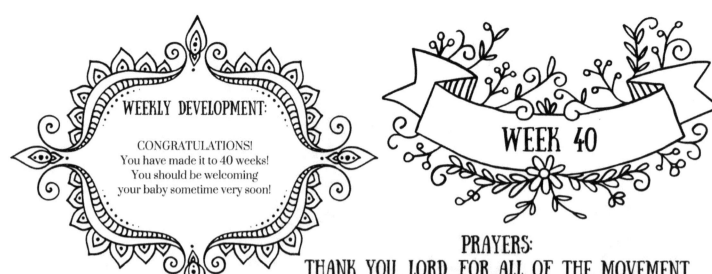

WEEKLY DEVELOPMENT:

CONGRATULATIONS!
You have made it to 40 weeks!
You should be welcoming
your baby sometime very soon!

WEEK 40

PRAYERS:
THANK YOU, LORD, FOR ALL OF THE MOVEMENT I HAVE BEEN BLESSED TO FEEL FROM THIS BABY. I PRAY THE MOVEMENTS CONTINUE AS THIS BABY GETS STRONGER AND READY TO MAKE HIS APPEARANCE.

GRACIOUS GOD, I AM SO THANKFUL I HAVE MADE IT TO FULL TERM WITH MY BABY. I KNOW YOU HAVE A PERFECT DELIVERY DATE, AND I REST IN YOUR PEACE AS THAT DAY APPROACHES.

TODAY I PRAY THAT MY BABY IS READY FOR DELIVERY AND THAT HE IS IN THE RIGHT POSITION, AND COMPLETELY READY TO COME OUT OF THE WOMB.

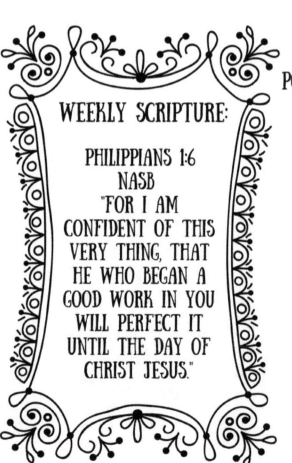

WEEKLY SCRIPTURE:

PHILIPPIANS 1:6
NASB
"FOR I AM CONFIDENT OF THIS VERY THING, THAT HE WHO BEGAN A GOOD WORK IN YOU WILL PERFECT IT UNTIL THE DAY OF CHRIST JESUS."

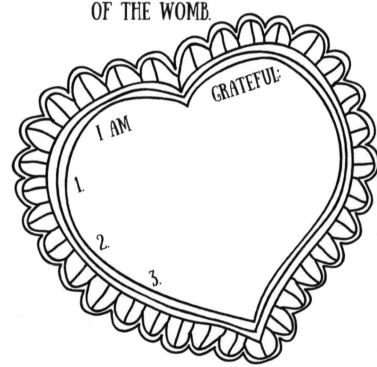

I AM GRATEFUL:

1.

2.

3.

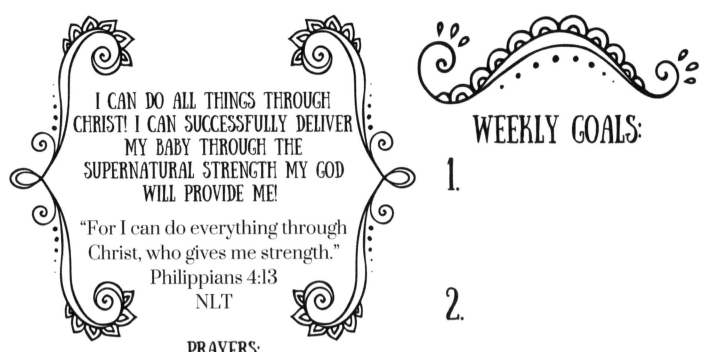

I CAN DO ALL THINGS THROUGH CHRIST! I CAN SUCCESSFULLY DELIVER MY BABY THROUGH THE SUPERNATURAL STRENGTH MY GOD WILL PROVIDE ME!

"For I can do everything through Christ, who gives me strength."
Philippians 4:13
NLT

WEEKLY GOALS:

1.

2.

3.

PRAYERS:

FATHER, I PRAY OVER MY RECOVERY TIME. I PRAY I WILL HAVE A SPEEDY RECOVERY THAT IS QUICK AND EASY.

TODAY I THANK YOU FOR A HEALTHY AND HAPPY BABY. I PRAY THE BABY WILL EASILY TRANSITION FROM THE WOMB TO THE WORLD.

LORD, I THANK YOU FOR A GOOD SLEEPER. I PRAY MY BABY WILL SLEEP EASILY AND PEACEFULLY AS HE GROWS AND MATURES OUT OF THE WOMB.

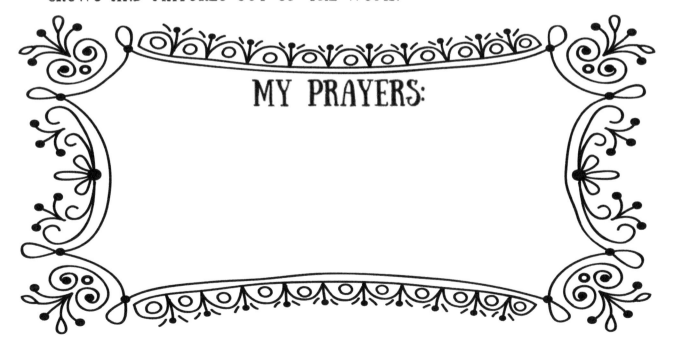

MY PRAYERS:

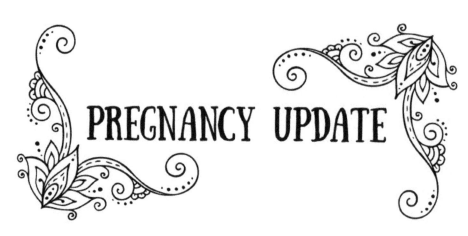

PREGNANCY UPDATE

OUR BIRTH STORY:

_____
_____
_____
_____

EMOTIONS I'M FEELING:

_____
_____
_____
_____

BIRTH STATS:

DATE & TIME:

_____
_____
_____

WEIGHT & LENGTH:

_____
_____

FAVORITE DELIVERY MEMORY:

_____
_____
_____

NOTES TO MY BABY:

_____
_____
_____
_____

NEWBORN PICTURE

CPSIA information can be obtained
at www.ICGtesting.com
Printed in the USA
BVHW07s0500270618
519767BV00001B/1/P